Understanding canine urinary incontinence

by Professor Peter Holt

Published by Vet Professionals

www.vetprofessionals.com

ISBN 978-0-9556913-9-3

About Dog Professional

Dog Professional is a subdivision of Vet Professionals Ltd. Dog Professional was founded in 2011 by Dr Sarah Caney with the aims of providing dog owners and veterinary professionals with the highest quality information, advice, training and consultancy services.

Publications

Dog Professional is a leading provider of high quality publications on caring for dogs with a variety of medical conditions. Written by international experts in their field, each book is written to be understood by care providers and veterinary professionals. The books are available to buy through the website www.dog-professional.com as eBooks where they can be downloaded and read instantly. Alternatively they can be purchased as a softback via the website and good bookstores. 'Understanding canine urinary incontinence' was first published in October 2011. 'Understanding canine diabetes mellitus' will be published later in 2011. A number of free to download articles and guides are also available on the Dog Professional website.

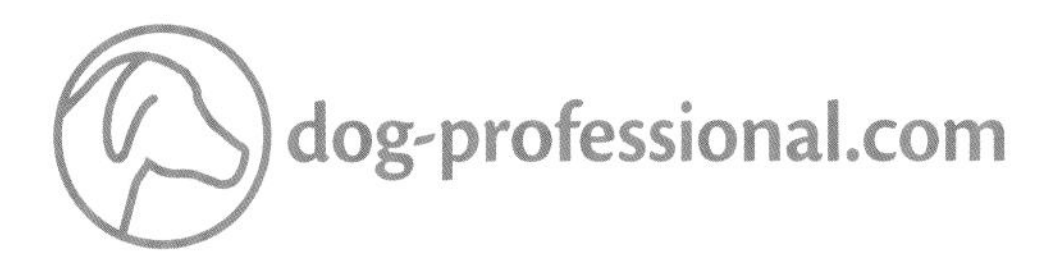

Advice, Training and Consultancy

Dog Professional is dedicated to improving the standards of canine care and in this capacity is a provider of Continuing Professional Development to veterinary surgeons, veterinary nurses and other professionals working with dogs around the world.

Dog Professional also works closely with leading providers of canine products and foods providing training programmes, assisting with product literature and advising on product design and marketing.

About the author

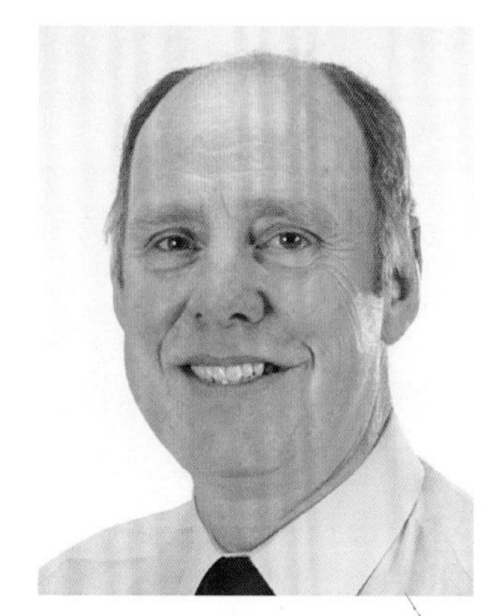

Peter Holt graduated from Glasgow University in 1970. After a year as House Surgeon there, he spent two years lecturing in small animal clinical studies in Nairobi, Kenya. A further seven years was spent in general practice before his appointment as lecturer at the University of Bristol where he was Professor of Veterinary Surgery until his retirement in 2009 when he was given the distinction of Emeritus Professor. His interests include aspects of soft tissue surgery, especially of the urinary system. He is author of, or contributor to, over 140 refereed papers and book chapters and has received six awards for his clinical and research activities. He has published two books on veterinary urology. He is a Past-President of the European Society of Veterinary Nephrology and Urology and in 1991 was awarded the Fellowship of the Royal College of Veterinary Surgeons for meritorious contributions to learning in the field of Veterinary Urology. In 2010, he was given Honorary Life Membership of the Association of Veterinary Soft Tissue Surgeons which has instituted an annual award in his name. The last 29 years of his career, he concentrated on the causes, investigation and treatment of urinary incontinence in small animals.

About this book

This book has been written as both a printed book and an interactive electronic book. Words in colour are contained in the **glossary section** at the end of the book.

Dedications and acknowledgements

This book is dedicated to the memory of Jill Jauncey, an outstanding breeder of beautiful Golden Retrievers and an even greater friend. Several dog-owning friends and relatives read the first draft of this book and I am particularly grateful to the following for their constructive comments: Sylvia Holt, Sharon and Andy Holt, Jane Vanstone and Brandon Turk, Barbara and Ken Stamp, Stella and Robin Dales, Margaret and Austin Chivers.

The pictures included in this book are the copyright of the author with the following exceptions which are produced by kind permission of those acknowledged:

Fig. 2 – this figure is reproduced by kind permission of Professor Dan Brockman.
Fig. 3a – thanks to Simon Bolton for providing the illustration on which this is based. This illustration is reproduced by kind permission of Vétoquinol.
Fig. 5 – this figure is reproduced by kind permission of the late Professor Harold Pearson.
Figs. 8, 11a-11f, 12a, 12c and 14 – are reproduced by kind permission of Manson Publishing Ltd.

CONTENTS

INTRODUCTION/FOREWORD

Urinary incontinence is a distressing complaint, not only for the dog but also for its owner (*Fig. 1*). There are no hard figures for the prevalence of canine urinary incontinence but it is seen commonly by veterinarians in general practice. Urinary incontinence is not a specific condition. Rather, it is a clinical sign recognised by the owner and for which there are a number of possible causes. These causes are discussed in more detail below and more space is given to the conditions which occur commonly than those which are rare.

This guide has been written to provide owners with the information they need, better to understand the complexities of urinary incontinence in dogs and its treatment. Veterinary scientific terms which might be difficult to understand are indicated in orange and linked to a glossary at the end of the book.

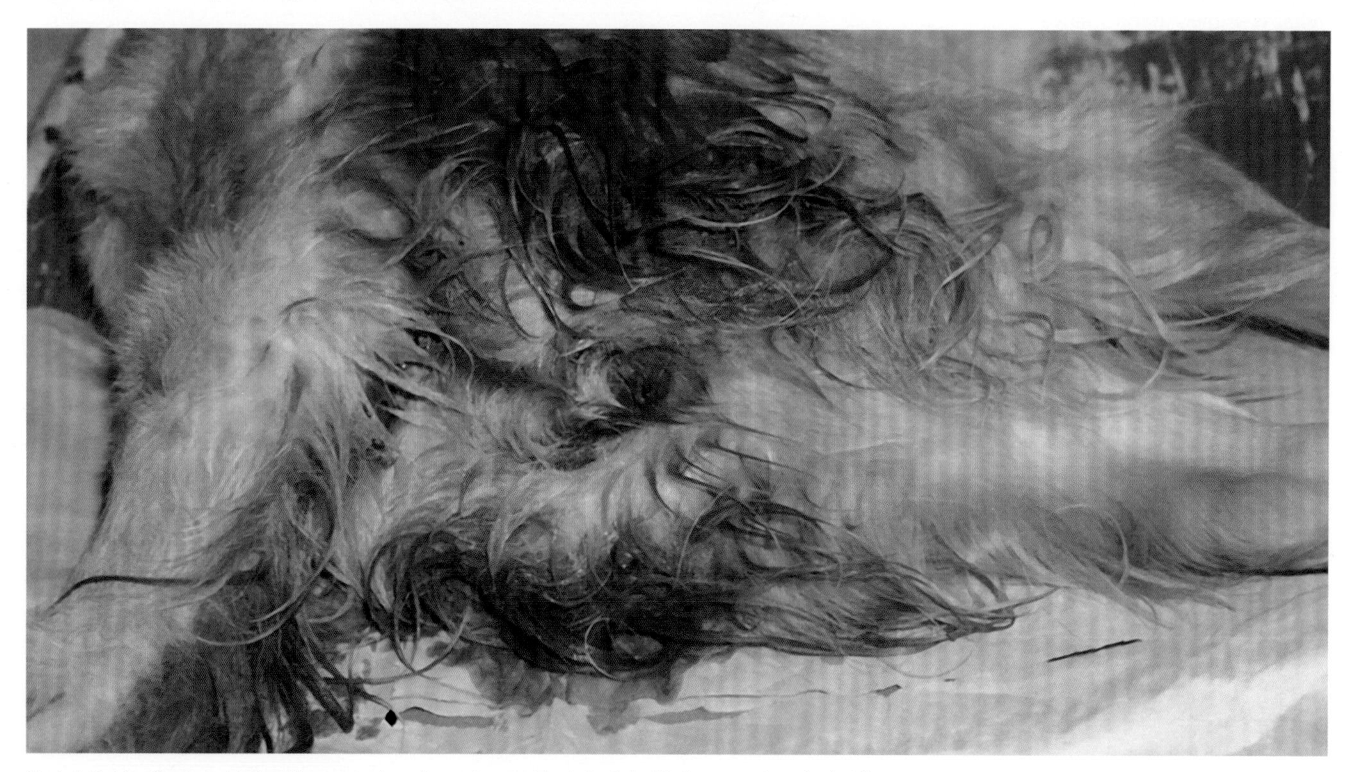

Fig. 1. A Golden Retriever bitch with severe urinary incontinence. The hair of the hind quarters is soaked with urine.

Realisation: coping with realising that you own an incontinent dog

When you first realise that your dog is incontinent, this may cause you some anxiety, especially if the condition progresses and worsens. In most cases, the incontinence is more of a problem to the owners than it is to the dog. Although the dog's skin will occasionally become scalded by the leaking urine, more often it is the unpleasant smell and wet dog bedding, carpets, chair upholstery and, if the dog sleeps there, owners' bedding that cause distress.

In most cases, the incontinence is more of a problem to the owners than it is to the dog.

The main problem with incontinence is the guilt many owners feel about their dog not leading a 'normal' life. The incontinence may be bad enough that some owners have to confine the dog to the kitchen or the garage to avoid the smell and damage urine causes to carpets etc. and because of health considerations for their children. The lengths some owners go to and their ingenuity are extraordinary (*Fig.* 2). The author had one client who plumbed the dog in, in the kitchen! The dog had a bed in the kitchen, the floor of which drained into a pipe which ran out through the kitchen wall, alongside that of the washing machine. Owners probably feel worse about confining their dog to certain areas than the dog itself does. Animals are remarkably adaptive and accepting of measures such as this, as long as they receive the usual love and attention provided by a caring owner. One of the joys of treating incontinence successfully is the fact that the dog can become more integrated into the household.

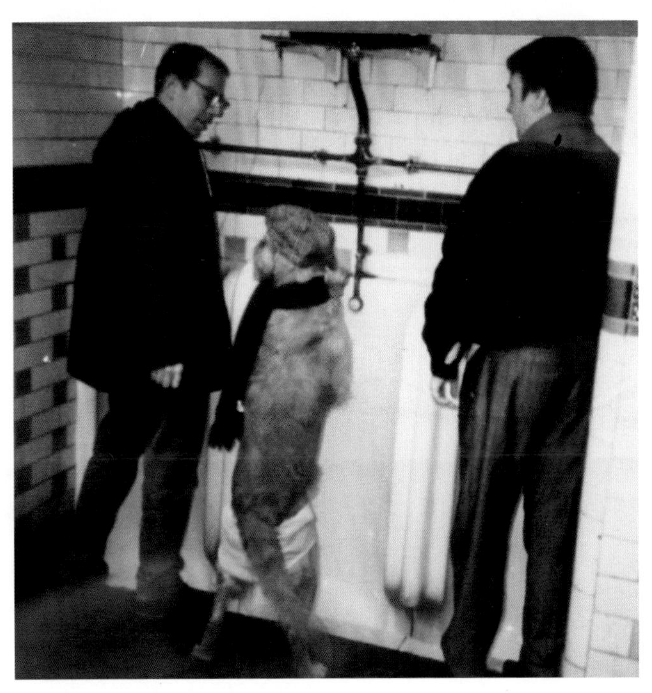

Fig. 2. Although this is a 'mock-up', the ingenuity some owners show in coping with an incontinent animal is extraordinary!

Another problem is conflict within the household. The author has been faced with couples arguing in his consulting room over their incontinent dog! One owner feels he/she cannot continue to afford replacement carpets, bedding (human and canine!) etc. and feels that euthanasia of the pet is the only option whilst the other feels they cannot condone putting an animal to sleep which is otherwise healthy. No-one is to blame in this situation; nothing the owners have done will have lead to the incontinence and nowadays, more can be done to investigate this clinical sign, find a cause for it and, in many cases, treat it successfully. It is extremely rare for the cause of the incontinence to be anything sinister, like cancer. The causes of incontinence and their treatment are discussed in more detail in **SECTION 2.**

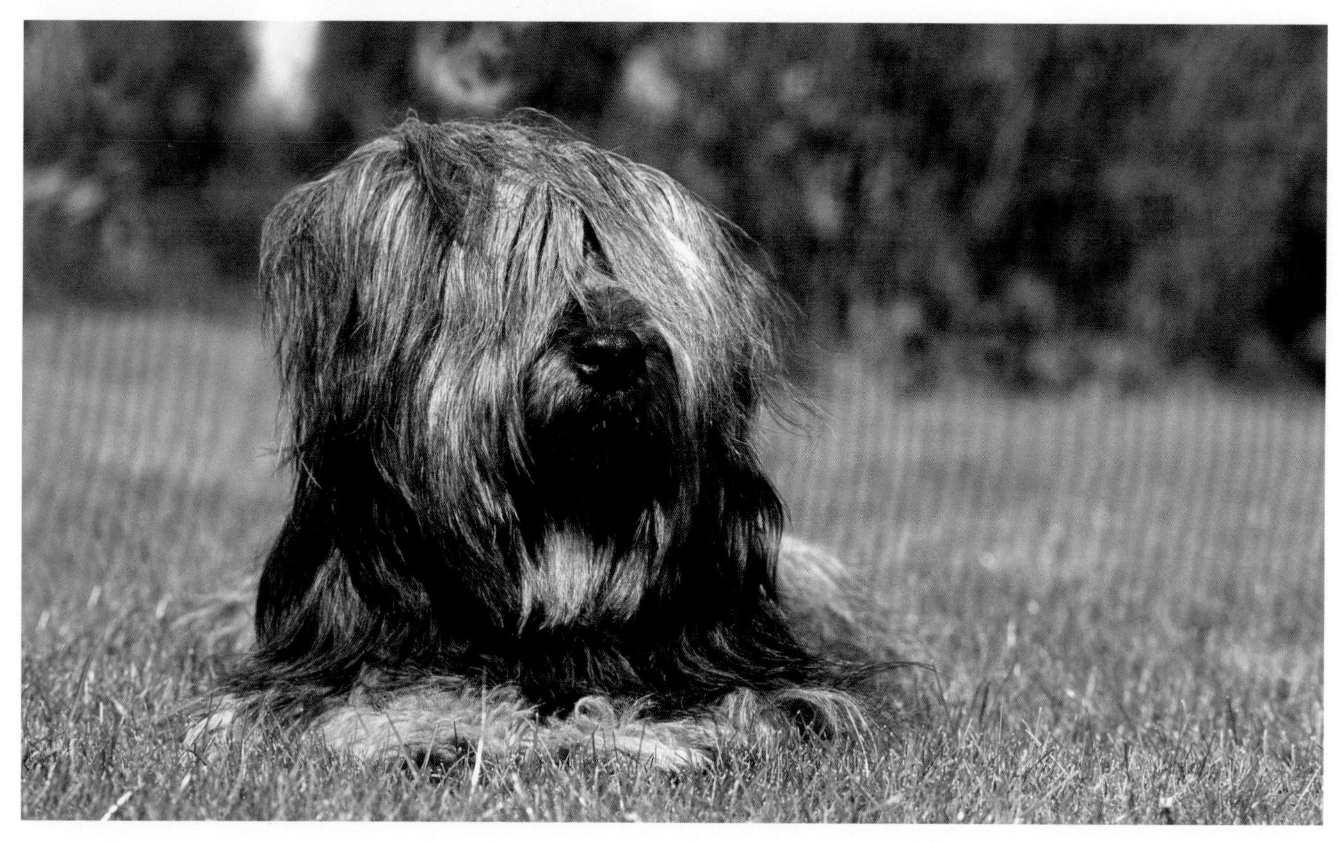

SECTION 2 | explaining the science of urinary incontinence

What is urinary incontinence?

Urinary incontinence is the passive leakage of urine over which the dog has no control. Most dogs with urinary incontinence will urinate normally but, in between urinations, will leak urine and this is detected by owners as damp patches, usually where the dog has been lying. Incontinence can occur at two main times of life. Juvenile incontinence is that which is present in puppies and has been noticed from birth (usually by the breeder) or since the puppy has been acquired by its first owner. More common, however, is acquired urinary incontinence which develops in a previously continent dog later in life.

What can genuine urinary incontinence be confused with?

Genuine, passive leakage of urine should not be confused with inadvertent urination or the dog which has a bladder irritation or drinks excessively and just 'has to go'. Inadvertent urination is not uncommon in puppies which get very excited when they greet their owners, to the extent that they wet themselves by passing urine uncontrollably. The good news is that most of these puppies grow out of this as they get older. Some dogs with severe bladder irritation – for example if they have cystitis – may feel an urgency to pass urine and urinate in the house if they cannot get outdoors in time or if the owners are out. The same is true of dogs which drink excessively and therefore have bladders which fill more quickly (any excessive thirst should be investigated by a veterinarian to rule out conditions like diabetes or kidney disease). This active urination in the house is not the same as passive, genuine incontinence.

Inadvertent urination is not uncommon in puppies which get very excited when they greet their owners

What problems does it cause the dog and its owners?

In most cases of incontinence, there are few problems for the dog itself, except in the *extremely* rare situation where the incontinence is related to a more serious condition such as cancer or severe spinal disease. In such cases, other, more severe signs are apparent such as difficulty urinating, increased urinary urgency and frequency, blood in the urine and difficulty in walking or even paraplegia (paralysis of the hindlimbs, usually caused by a spinal problem).

How is continence controlled normally and how might this control be lost?

To understand this, we must first review the anatomy of the urinary tract. This is summarised in *Fig. 3* on page 10. Urine is produced by the kidneys and passes down fine tubes, the ureters, into the urinary bladder. In a continent animal, urine entering the bladder is stored there until it is convenient for the dog to pass it. Normal urine storage in the bladder depends on a bladder which can gradually fill with urine without a marked increase in pressure within the bladder and a tight 'sphincter' to

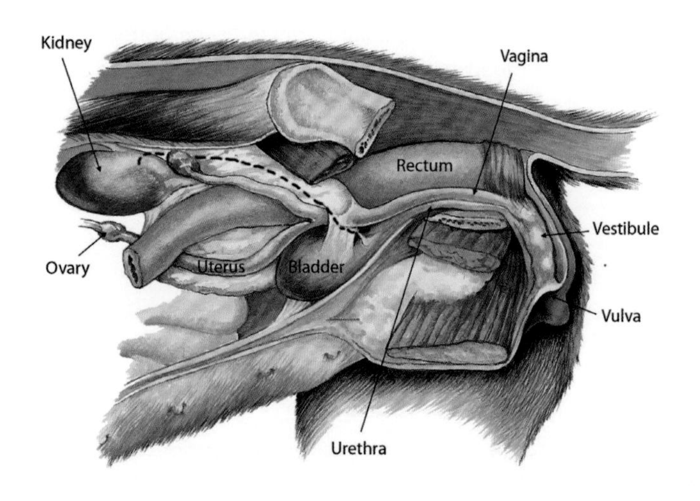

keep the bladder outlet closed and the urine in. In fact, the whole of the tube leading from the bladder to the outside (the urethra) is a tube of resistance which contributes to the 'sphincter'. It is composed of muscle (both striated muscle, over which the animal has control and smooth muscle which can maintain tone without voluntary control). However, a number of other factors besides muscle contribute to the resistance in the tube and these are summarised in the section covering Acquired Urethral Sphincter Mechanism Incompetence. The muscles of the bladder and the urethra are supplied by nerves. Those to the bladder result in relaxation of the bladder during urine storage (so it fills without much increase in pressure within the bladder) and contraction during urination in order to empty the bladder. The nerves to the urethral muscles maintain tone during storage of urine (to keep the bladder outlet closed) and relax when the dog is urinating to allow the urethra to open so urine can flow out.

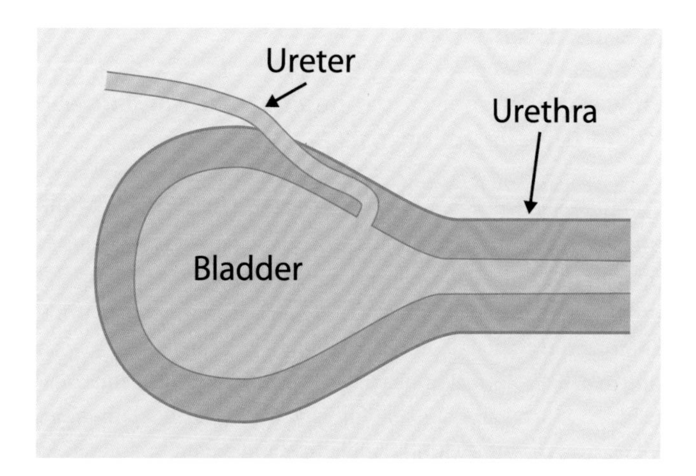

Fig. 3a (top). The basic anatomy of the urinary tract of the bitch, as seen from the animal's left hand side. Urine produced by the kidney (there are usually two but only one is shown here) passes down a fine tube, the ureter, into the bladder. The ureter is covered in fat and so cannot be seen but its course is indicated by the broken black line. Urine is stored in the bladder until the dog wishes to urinate. During urination, urine passes down the urethra and out via the vestibule and vulva in the bitch. In the male dog, the urethra is much longer and curves around the back of the pelvic floor into the penis where it opens (see *Fig. 13 on* page 23). Note that the ureter passes through the bladder wall for a short distance before opening into it (*Fig. 3b, left*). This is so that, when the bladder contracts during urination, this section of the ureter is compressed and closes, preventing urine passing the wrong way, back up the ureter.

Bearing all this in mind, for urinary incontinence to occur, at least one of the following must be happening (examples of specific conditions leading to this are given in brackets):

- The pressure within the bladder is normal but the resistance of the urethra is too low to prevent urine leakage, especially if any extra pressure acts to squeeze the bladder (see sections on **Congenital** and **Acquired Urethral Sphincter Mechanism Incompetence**).
- The resistance of the urethra is normal but the pressure in the bladder is too high and exceeds this resistance (see section on **Detrusor Overactivity/Instability**).
- The pressure within the bladder and the resistance of the urethra are normal but urine outflow by-passes the urethral sphincter mechanism (see section on **Ectopic Ureter**).

What are the causes of urinary incontinence in juvenile animals?

Genuine urinary incontinence is rare in puppies. To put this in perspective, ectopic ureter, the commonest cause of urinary incontinence in juvenile dogs, was only seen once by the author during his seven years in small animal practice.

The list of possible causes of juvenile urinary incontinence is:

- Ectopic ureter
- Congenital urethral sphincter mechanism incompetence
- Bladder hypoplasia

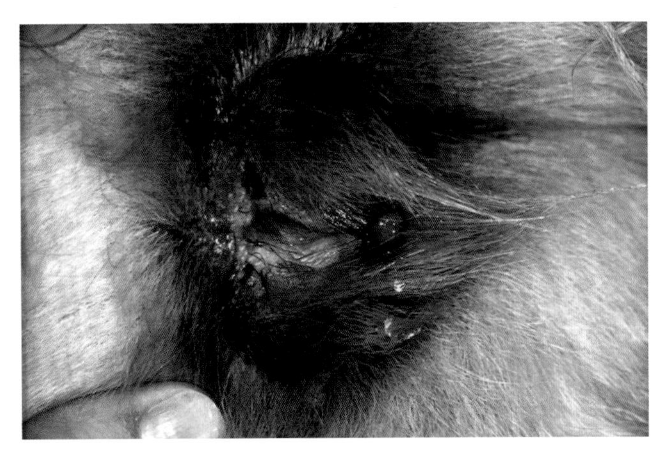

Fig. 4. This Golden Retriever bitch with an ectopic-ureter is dripping urine continuously.

- Pervious urachus
- Intersexuality
- Congenital neurological problems

Ectopic Ureter

Although rare, this is the commonest cause of urinary incontinence in juvenile dogs (44% of incontinent juvenile dogs). This is mainly a problem of dogs but has also been reported in cats, horses and cattle. Dogs with this condition are born with one, or sometimes both, ureters failing to open into the bladder. Instead, the ureters open further down the urinary tract (compare *Fig. 3b* on page 10 with *Fig. 15*, left diagram on page 24). Thus urine, instead of going into the bladder to be stored, passes into the urethra or sometimes the vagina (of bitches) and so most of these puppies show continuous leakage of urine. Ectopic ureter is much more common in female than male animals. There is a breed predisposition in the UK (Labradors, Golden Retrievers and Skye terriers) whilst in the USA Siberian Huskies, Newfoundlands, Bulldogs, West Highland White terriers, Fox terriers and Miniature and Toy Poodles appear to be at risk.

The cause is unknown but hereditary factors may play a role. Incontinence may be continuous (*Fig. 4,* page 11) or intermittent and even when both ureters are ectopic (bilateral ectopic ureter), the dog can usually still pass a normal stream of urine, despite the copious leakage at other times. Diagnosis is by contrast radiography (special x-ray studies discussed in more detail in the section **How is urinary incontinence investigated?**). Secondary complications are common and usually involve the kidney and ureter on the affected side. For example, the area of the kidney where urine collects before passing down the ureter may become dilated (distended) with urine (hydronephrosis) or infected (pyelonephritis) and the ectopic ureter itself is usually dilated with urine (hydro-ureter).

Congenital Urethral Sphincter Mechanism Incompetence

Congenital urethral sphincter mechanism incompetence means that the dog is born with a weakness of the urethral sphincter mechanism. This is the second most common cause of juvenile incontinence (35% of incontinent juvenile dogs) and tends to be a problem of large breeds of dog, predominantly bitches. Leakage of urine is more copious compared to animals with ectopic ureters and occurs predominantly when the dogs are lying down and relaxed or asleep. The urethra may be abnormally short (urethral hypoplasia) or even absent. Urethral diverticula (cavities outpouching from the urethra) and urethral dilatations may be present in male animals.

In many bitches, no gross abnormalities are detected on contrast radiography, apart from a bladder which is located too far back ('caudally positioned bladder') and the diagnosis frequently relies on the history and elimination of other possible causes of incontinence. Urodynamic investigations (such as a technique called urethral pressure profilometry) can be used to measure the resistance in the urethra and are of some value but are not always diagnostic and are rarely available in most veterinary practices.

Bladder Hypoplasia

Bladder hypoplasia basically means that the dog has been born with a bladder which is too small for the size of the animal. This is a subjective diagnosis and it is unclear if the problem is true bladder hypoplasia or failure of normal bladder growth and development. It is commonly associated with other congenital (present from birth) causes of incontinence but may, rarely, occur alone. The diagnosis is confirmed by contrast radiography as only a small amount of contrast medium is required to fill the bladder during retrograde techniques (see later). It is important in animals with a presumptive diagnosis of bladder hypoplasia to eliminate other causes of incontinence which may also be present. For example, the small bladder may be a reflection of poor bladder development because of lack of stimulation by adequate volumes of urine in the bladder (e.g. the dog with ectopic ureter in which much of the urine bypasses the bladder and so is not stored).

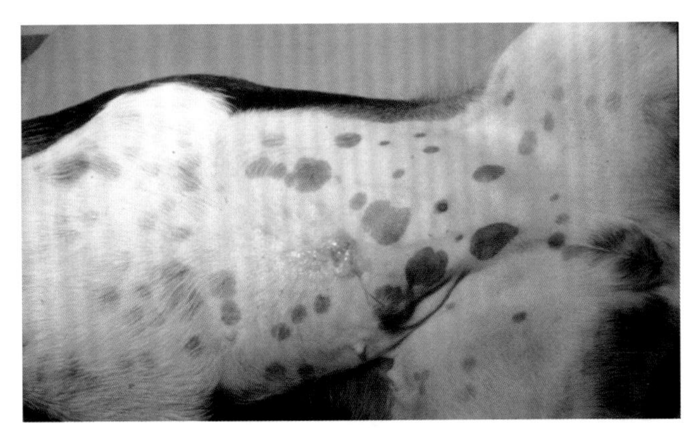

Fig. 5. In pervious urachus, leakage of urine is via the umbilicus and may result in local skin scalding, as can be seen in this beagle puppy.

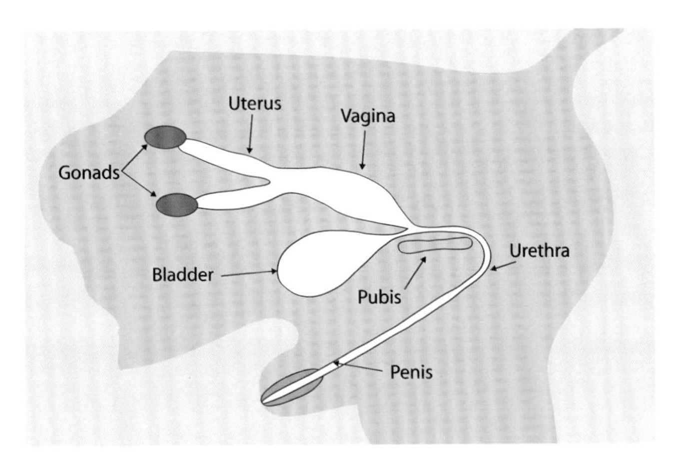

Fig. 6. Diagrammatic representation of the commonest anatomical abnormalities present in intersex dogs which are incontinent. Although these dogs have a male type of lower urinary tract anatomy, they also have a vagina which opens into the urethra. When they urinate, some of the urine passes from the urethra into this vagina. In between urinations, the urine in the vagina may leak out, leading to the sign of incontinence.

Pervious Urachus

Pervious urachus is seen when a communication (the urachus), which is present in the foetus, between the bladder and the umbilicus (navel) fails to close before birth. This means that the leakage of urine occurs through the umbilicus, leading to scalding of the skin on the lower abdomen in that region (*Fig.* 5). It is very rare in puppies compared to horses and farm animals. This condition is easily diagnosed since incontinence occurs through the umbilicus which may be scalded with urine. Contrast radiography confirms the diagnosis (see later).

Intersexuality

Intersexuality occurs when animals are born with both male and female genitalia. Rarely, intersex animals may be incontinent. During urination, some of the urine passes normally down the urethra while some urine accumulates in abnormally-present internal sex organs (for example within a vagina inside a dog which externally looks male! – *Fig.* 6). The urine which accumulates in the vagina subsequently leaks out via the urethra between urinations, thus leading to the sign of incontinence. Diagnosis relies on contrast radiography such as retrograde positive contrast urethrocystography (contrast imaging of the urethra and bladder).

Congenital Neurological Conditions

Very rarely, puppies are born with abnormalities of the spine. The main sign in these animals is an inability to stand and/or walk normally but incontinence (urinary and faecal) may also be present. Spinal radiography and or MRI scanning may confirm the diagnosis.

What are the causes of urinary incontinence in adult animals?

Most causes of urinary incontinence in dogs are acquired; that is, they develop in adulthood in a dog which was previously continent. Incontinence in adults is *much* more common in bitches than in male dogs. Although there are many conditions which can lead to urinary incontinence in adults, by far the commonest (80% of incontinent adult bitches) is acquired urethral sphincter mechanism incompetence. More details will be given about this condition than the other, much rarer, causes of incontinence therefore. The main causes of adult incontinence are:

- Acquired urethral sphincter mechanism incompetence
- Prostatic diseases
- Bladder neoplasia (cancer)
- Ureterovaginal fistula
- Acquired neurological conditions
- 'Overflow' incontinence
- Detrusor overactivity/instability

Acquired Urethral Sphincter Mechanism Incompetence

In adult dogs referred for the investigation of urinary incontinence, urethral sphincter mechanism incompetence – failure of the urethral sphincter mechanism – is by far the commonest diagnosis made, affecting 80% of incontinent bitches. In these animals, incontinence occurs mainly when the dogs are recumbent and relaxed (*Fig. 7*). Although this is the doggy equivalent of human stress incontinence, few of these animals leak doing aerobics! Thus most owners notice that there

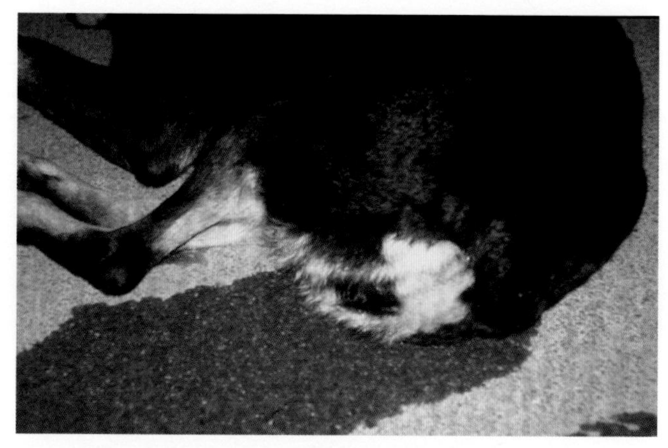

Fig. 7. Urine leakage in an adult Rottweiler bitch with acquired urethral sphincter mechanism incompetence. In adult female and male dogs with this problem, urine leakage occurs predominantly when the dogs are lying down and relaxed.

are damp patches or pools of urine on the floor, carpets etc. where the dog has been lying. Although urethral pressure profilometry – measurement of the tone of the urethral wall – can be used to demonstrate incompetence of the urethral sphincter mechanism, this technique is not readily available in general practice and is predisposed to a number of artefacts which can make interpretation difficult. In general practice, therefore, the diagnosis is usually made on the basis of the breed, history and by the elimination of other possible diagnoses using imaging (radiography) and laboratory techniques. Acquired urethral sphincter mechanism incompetence usually (but not always) follows neutering in both bitches and male dogs. Before treatment can be contemplated, an understanding of the pathophysiology (i.e. the factors which contribute to the condition) of urethral sphincter mechanism incompetence is required. Our current knowledge is more extensive in the bitch (the commonest sex affected) and so what follows relates to female dogs although mention will be made of males later. Since no true bladder neck sphincter muscle exists in the bitch and continence is maintained by a complex mechanism of interacting factors, the term 'urethral sphincter mechanism incompetence' has been used to describe a weakness of urinary continence control.

The 'urethral sphincter mechanism' is a term used to summarise the forces acting in the urethra to keep the urethra closed and prevent incontinence. A number of factors are believed to contribute towards this sphincter mechanism and these include:

- Urethral tone – the ability of the tissues of the urethral wall to prevent the passage of urine when an animal is not urinating. Measurement of urethral tone (urethral pressure profilometry) has demonstrated that poor urethral tone is implicated in urinary incontinence. Urethral tone is maintained by a complex interaction of neuromuscular, vascular and passive elastic components and it is unclear which of these is deficient in sphincter mechanism incompetence.

- Length of the urethra – there is considerable variation in urethral length between bitches of different sizes. However, taking body size into consideration, bitches with sphincter mechanism incompetence tend to have shorter urethras than continent animals.

- Position of the bladder neck – a number of authors recorded the radiographic finding of a caudally positioned bladder (also referred to as a 'pelvic bladder') during the investigation of incontinent animals (compare *Fig. 12c* with *Fig. 12a* on page 22). The significance of this finding was disputed in the past but there is now good evidence that an intrapelvic bladder neck (i.e. a bladder the neck of which is too far back, inside the pelvic cavity – a so-called 'pelvic bladder') contributes significantly to urinary incontinence due to urethral sphincter mechanism incompetence. The caudal bladder position in affected dogs is associated with the shorter urethral length and also the fact that the bladder moves backwards when a bitch moves from a standing to a relaxed recumbent position. This movement is more pronounced in bitches with urethral sphincter mechanism incompetence than in continent animals, suggesting a deficiency in supporting mechanisms in the lower urinary tract of affected animals.

- Breed and body size – body size appears to be a factor since large and giant breeds are particularly at risk. Urethral sphincter mechanism incompetence is most common in the UK in Dobermans and Old English Sheepdogs, and there is evidence that these breeds and Rottweilers, Weimaraners, Springer Spaniels and Irish Setters are at increased risk for developing this form of incontinence.

- Obesity – whilst not a cause of the condition, obesity may worsen the degree of incontinence.

- Neutering and hormones – there is an association between neutering (spaying) and urinary incontinence and this is probably due to a lack of circulating oestrogens or an excess of other hormones which are not suppressed after neutering. In general terms, spayed animals are nearly eight times as likely to develop this form of urinary incontinence than entire bitches. This sounds quite scary until you put it into perspective. If you did not neuter 100 bitches and observed them for 10 years, two would become incontinent in that period. If you took 100 bitches and did neuter them, by 10 years later 16 of them would be incontinent. So, although there is an eight fold increase in the incidence, 84 of the bitches neutered 10 years previously would still be bone dry! This risk has to be balanced against the benefits of neutering bitches such as reducing the risk of mammary cancer, eliminating the risk of ovarian cancer and eliminating the risk of pyometra (a serious condition of the womb that can develop in entire bitches). Spaying before the first season may increase the risk of development of urinary incontinence although this has yet to be proved conclusively.

The exact abnormality leading to urethral sphincter mechanism incompetence and the region of the urethra in which it occurs are unknown. It is a multi-factorial problem and a variety of factors – as listed above – may contribute to causing incontinence in any individual.

Urethral sphincter mechanism incompetence in male dogs is uncommon. As in the bitch, the acquired form often follows neutering and larger breeds appear to be at risk. Also like the situation in bitches, incontinence is likely to occur when intra-abdominal pressure increases (e.g. when lying down and relaxed/asleep) and affected animals tend to have caudally positioned bladder necks, although a short urethra does not appear to be a factor in males.

Prostatic Disease

The prostate gland surrounds the urethra near the neck of the bladder in male dogs (bitches do not have a prostate gland) and so its enlargement or inflammation can have an effect on urethral function and thus bladder emptying or continence control. Although incontinence can occur rarely in male dogs with prostate diseases, such dogs are far more likely to exhibit other signs such as bloody urine (haematuria) and difficulty passing urine (dysuria) and faeces. There are a large number of conditions which can affect the canine prostate gland. Most of these are benign and treatable but prostate cancer can also occur, albeit rarely, in dogs.

Bladder Neoplasia

Sometimes, animals with bladder tumours can be incontinent. This is extremely rare but, when it does occur, is more often associated with malignant bladder cancers. Most dogs with bladder cancer are presented with other signs such as urgency to urinate, increased frequency of urination and/or blood in the urine (haematuria). It is not clear what leads to the incontinence in these rare cases. It is likely that incontinent dogs with bladder neck/urethral neoplasia have impairment of the sphincter mechanism whereas bladder wall tumours probably result in detrusor instability (see later).

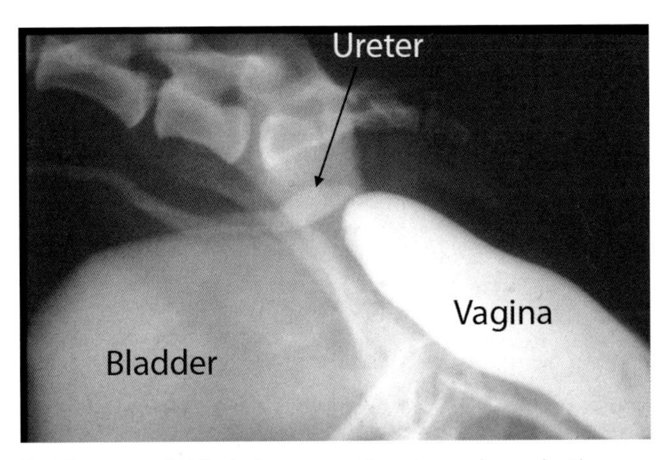

Fig. 8. A ureterovaginal fistula demonstrated by vagino-urethrography. The contrast medium which has been introduced into the vagina has passed down the urethra and into the bladder, as expected. However, some contrast medium can be seen passing into a ureter which opens abnormally into the vagina.

Diagnosis is confirmed by contrast radiography (urethrocystography – contrast imaging of the bladder and urethra) and/or ultrasonography but, because of the possibility of malignancy, examinations to check for spread of any tumour (such as x-rays of the chest and abdomen) should also be carried out. Even in the absence of evidence of any spread, histopathological examination of a biopsy of the mass or the excised tumour is essential to obtain a prognosis.

Ureterovaginal Fistula

This is an extremely rare complication of spaying (neutering a female) and probably results from inadvertent inclusion of a ureter during tying off (ligation) of the cranial vagina or because of adhesions between the ureter and the vagina. The ureter can form a fistula (an abnormal passageway) into the vagina and so an acquired ectopic ureter draining into the vagina results and can be diagnosed by contrast radiography (*Fig. 8*). Even rarer in dogs is vesicovaginal fistulation where a fistula develops between the bladder and vagina, leading to incontinence. This is also reported occasionally in women after gynaecological surgery.

Acquired Neurological Conditions

As with congenital neurological conditions, acquired urinary retention with overflow incontinence may result from neurological dysfunction, usually as a sequel to spinal lesions (e.g. intervertebral disc prolapse, tumours). Here, the impaired nerve supply means that the bladder cannot empty and so urine builds up in it. Eventually, the pressure in the bladder overcomes the urethral resistance and urine leakage occurs. Other neurological abnormalities such as paraplegia are usually apparent and the diagnosis may be confirmed by radiography or advanced imaging such as MRI or CT scanning.

Overflow Incontinence with Chronic Retention

Animals with urinary obstruction, for example caused by urethral calculi (stones) or tumours may, paradoxically, become incontinent when the pressure of urine building up within the bladder (the intravesical pressure) becomes high enough to overcome the urethral resistance. Such cases are primarily presented with dysuria and should be investigated and treated as such.

Detrusor Overactivity/Instability

In these cases, uncontrollable bladder contractions occur, resulting in voiding of urine. In dogs, detrusor instability is often secondary to conditions leading to excessive bladder wall stimulation (e.g. cystitis, bladder tumours). Such stimulation may also occur in juvenile animals with bladder hypoplasia, especially if they are housed for long periods (e.g. overnight) and unable to inhibit the detrusor reflex. The owners of such animals may report nocturia or marked bed-wetting overnight.

Occasionally, as in man, detrusor overactivity occurs with no obvious underlying cause. It may be present alone or (rarely) in conjunction with urethral sphincter mechanism incompetence. Diagnosis depends upon the taking of a detailed history and elimination of other causes of incontinence. In humans, this condition is diagnosed using cystometric studies (measurements of pressures within the bladder and/or urethra) but this requires great patient co-operation, something we do not have with our canine patients!

How is urinary incontinence investigated?

A wide variety of techniques are used to determine the cause of urinary incontinence in dogs. These start with the taking of a good history (see **Section 4** for how you can help with this). This is usually followed by clinical examination (*Fig. 9*). Since there are few abnormalities which can be detected clinically in most incontinent dogs (apart from evidence of incontinence – *Fig. 10*), the history often gives more of a clue to the cause than the clinical examination does. Thus, a juvenile Golden Retriever which has leaked urine continuously since it was born is likely to have ectopic ureter(s). In contrast, a Doberman bitch which was continent as a juvenile but has developed incontinence since it was spayed and which occurs mainly when it is lying down and relaxed/asleep is likely to have acquired urethral sphincter

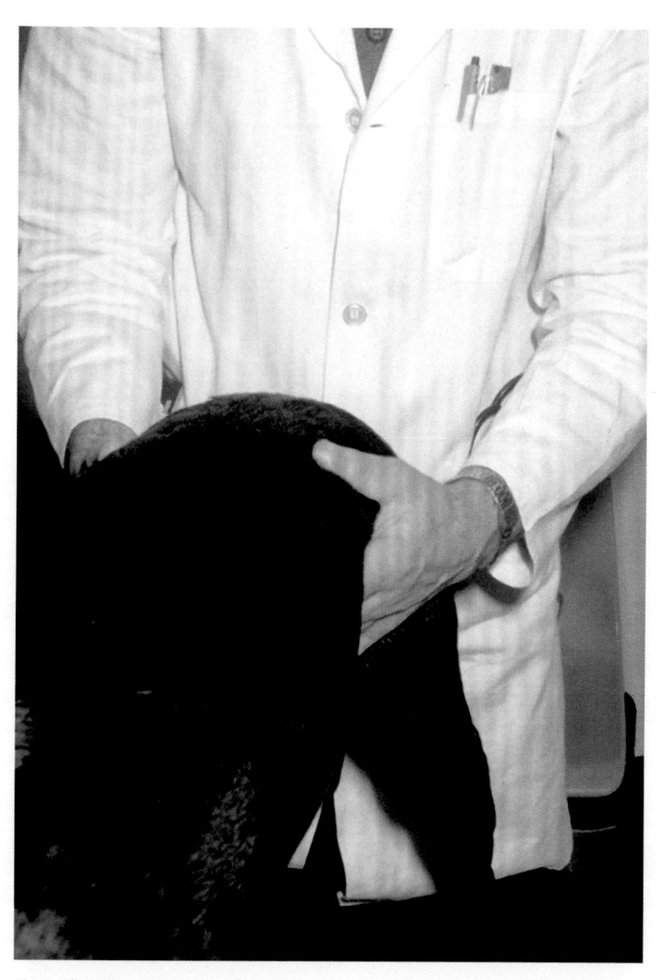

Fig. 9. Clinical examination of the kidneys is possible in some dogs like this co-operative, relaxed Labrador but can be difficult, if not impossible, in tense and/or overweight dogs. In most incontinent animals, there is often little to detect on clinical examinations alone.

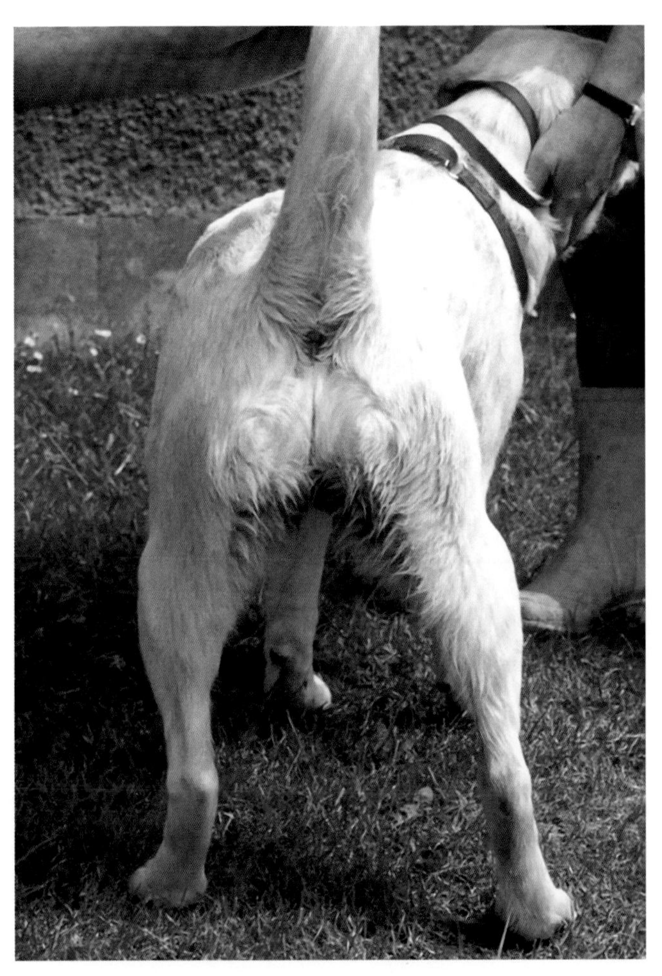

Fig. 10. In this Labrador bitch with an ectopic ureter, the urine leakage is obvious during clinical examinations.

mechanism incompetence. However, the history is not foolproof and more detailed investigations are required to confirm a suspected diagnosis and rule out other possibilities. These investigations include blood and urine laboratory work and using methods of visualising the urinary tract. Although the latter can include passing endoscopes into the urinary tract and even MRI or CT scanning, in the vast majority of cases, contrast radiography is sufficient to reach a diagnosis and is readily available in almost all veterinary practices. Contrast radiography has to be used because the details of the urinary tract are not visible on normal radiographs. During contrast radiography, a liquid which shows up white on radiographs (contrast medium) is introduced into the urinary tract. To show up the kidneys and ureters, the contrast medium is injected into a vein from where it travels via the blood circulation to the kidneys where it is excreted. This is called intravenous urography (*Fig. 11* on pages 20 and 21). To demonstrate the lower urinary tract, contrast medium is introduced into the vagina of the bitch, from where it flows into the urethra and bladder (vagino-urethrography) (*Fig. 12* on page 22). In male dogs, contrast medium is introduced directly into the urethra (urethrocystography) (*Fig. 13* on page 23). Sometimes in the bladder, air is used as a contrast medium. A general anaesthetic is required for these investigations. Apart from eliminating the possibility of any movement or discomfort or stress caused by the techniques used, it also prevents artefacts which can be seen if some of these techniques are performed in the conscious animal. Sometimes ultrasonography of the urinary tract of incontinent animals is performed and is useful for assessing the physical state of the kidneys (*Fig. 14* on page 23), prostate and other urinary organs.

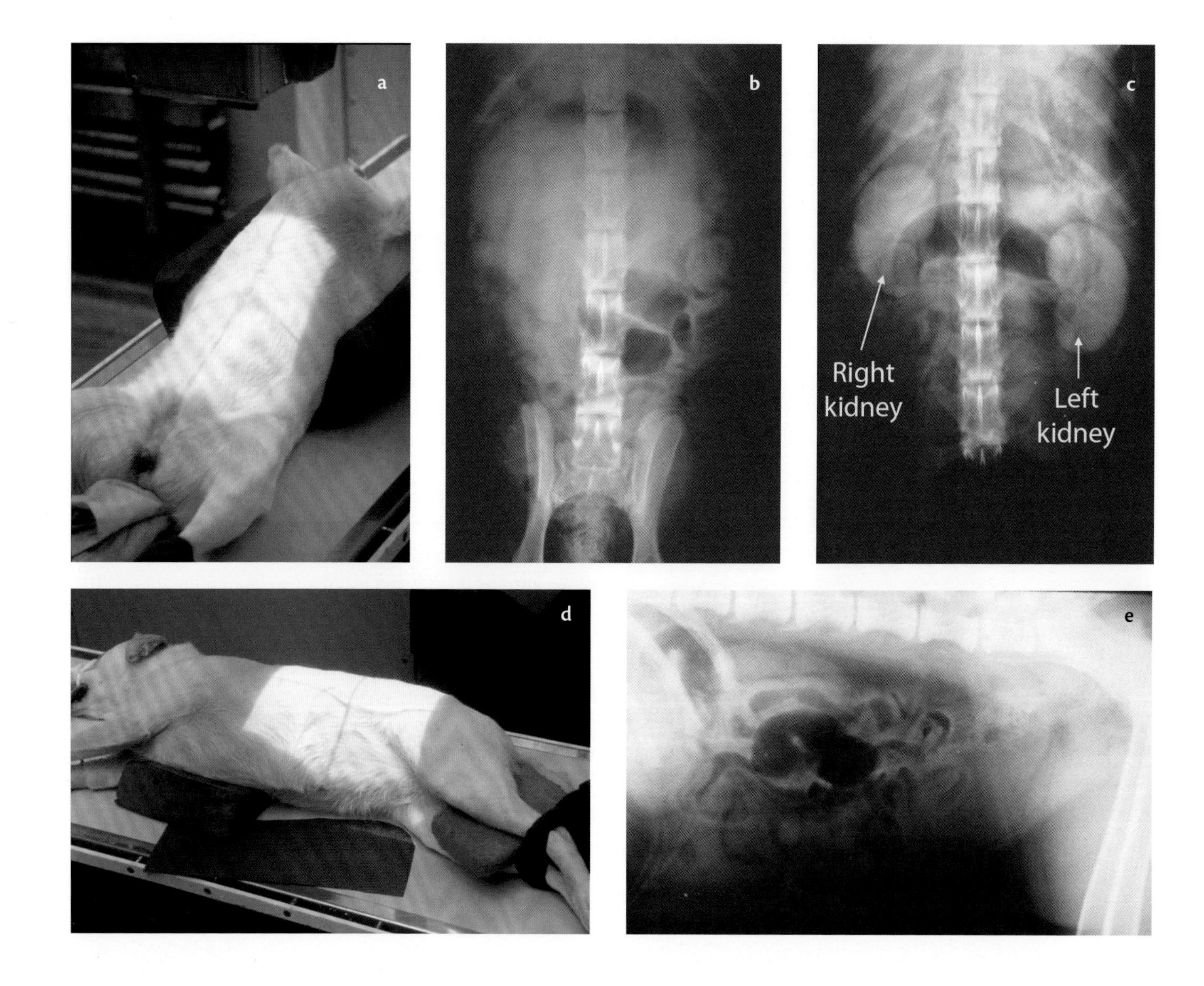
a
b
c
Right kidney
Left kidney
d
e

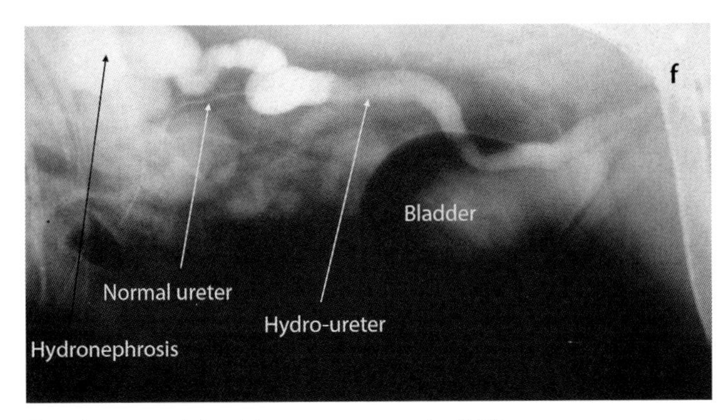

Fig. 11 (page 20 and above). Intravenous urography (IVU):

a. The patient has been positioned so that the X-ray beam passes from the front to the back of the abdomen (a 'ventrodorsal' view).

b. Before any contrast medium is given, an X-ray is taken (the 'control' or 'plain' film). This is to make sure that the exposure is correct and that there is nothing in the abdomen which may make later films difficult to read (e.g. lots of faeces in the intestine!). However, note that it is difficult to see any urinary tract anatomy. This is not abnormal; it is always difficult to see any details, hence the need for the contrast medium.

c. Compare this film with Fig. 11b. This X-ray was taken just after contrast medium was injected into a vein. The contrast medium has passed via the circulation to the kidneys which are now showing up nicely. These kidneys look normal (note that it is normal for the right kidney to be higher up in the abdomen than the left). When looking at X-rays, 'left' and 'right' refer to the animal's left and right and not how they appear when you are looking at the x-ray.

d. During the examination, the dog is positioned for side views (the so-called 'lateral' views) of the abdomen.

e. Again, the plain lateral view (taken at the beginning of the study before any contrast medium is given) reveals little urinary tract anatomy.

f. Compare this film with Fig. 11e. This was taken later in an IVU of an incontinent dog and shows a dilated collecting area in the right kidney (hydronephrosis) and a dilated right ureter (hydro-ureter) which is missing the bladder out and opening lower down the urinary tract (i.e. an ectopic ureter). The normal (left) ureter is arrowed for comparison.

What are the options for treating urinary incontinence?

Juvenile incontinence

Ectopic ureters – treatment of ectopic ureters involves transplanting the ureter into the bladder or removal of the ureter and associated kidney if severe secondary disease is present and only one of the two kidneys is affected. Transplantation techniques nowadays usually involve intravesical stomatisation of the intramural ectopic ureter (which most are) followed by occlusion or removal of the ureter beyond the stoma (illustrated diagrammatically in *Fig. 15* on page 24). If both your dog's ureters are ectopic, it may not be possible to operate on them at the same time. During surgery, the bladder wall in the region of the new ureter opening swells (especially in puppies – this is one of the reasons why surgery may be postponed until the dog is at least 4-5 months old, since swelling is less likely in older animals). This swelling can sometimes be severe enough to temporarily block the new ureter opening. This is usually not a problem because the other kidney and its ureter are able to cope with urine output until the swelling settles down and the transplanted ureter opens up again. However, if surgery is performed on both ureters and swelling occurs, this can have serious consequences. Most surgeons therefore transplant one ureter and assess the degree of bladder wall swelling at the time of surgery to decide if they think it is safe to proceed with transplantation of the second ureter during the same operation or not. If not, the second ureter is usually transplanted 4-8 weeks later. Sometimes, this swelling can involve the neck of the bladder and make it difficult for the dog to pass urine for a few days until it settles down, but this is rare.

Congenital urethral sphincter mechanism incompetence – approximately half of juvenile bitches with congenital urethral sphincter mechanism incompetence will become continent after their first or second season (and so should not be spayed before then). Oestrogens should also not be used to treat juvenile bitches with this condition because of possible adverse 'feed-back' effects on the pituitary gland. These may have the effect of suppressing oestrus, something we want to take place in incontinent juvenile bitches. However, alpha-adrenergics such as phenylpropanolamine (Propalin, Vétoquinol; Urilin, Dechra Veterinary Products) and ephedrine (Enurace, Elanco Animal Health) could be used to stimulate the smooth muscle of the urethra and may improve the situation whilst oestrus and its effects on continence control are awaited. Similarly, a few male dogs improve after puberty. Those animals that do not may be candidates for medical or surgical management. In bitches, management with alpha-adrenergics may be continued or

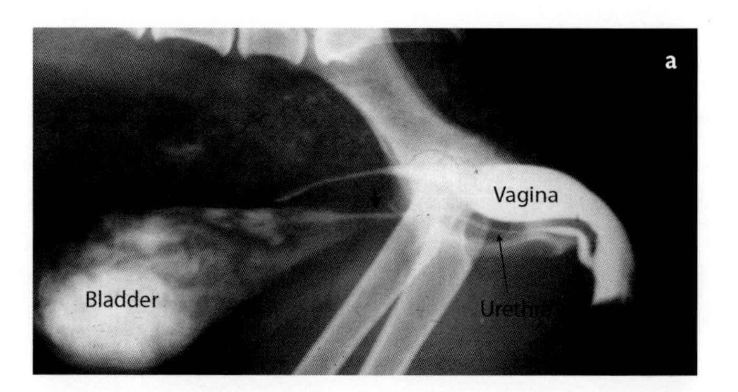

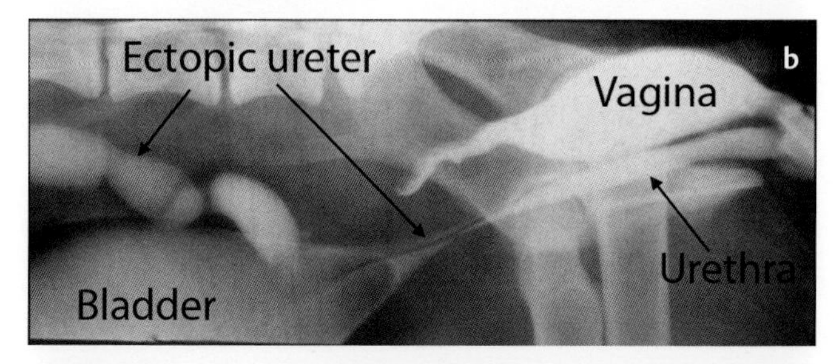

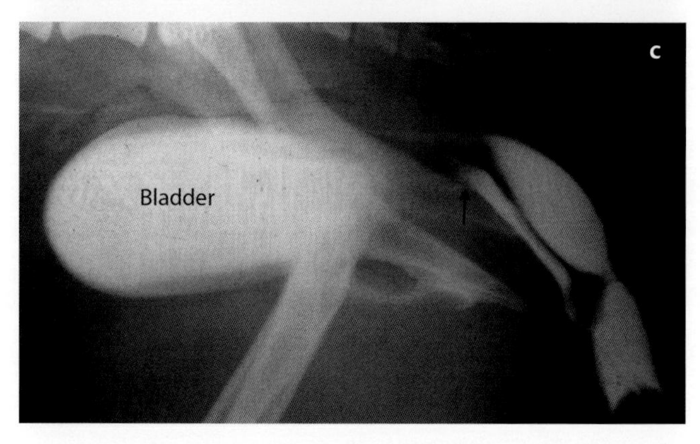

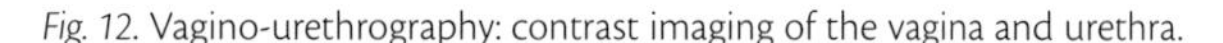

Fig. 12. Vagino-urethrography: contrast imaging of the vagina and urethra.

a. During vagino-urethrography, contrast medium is introduced into the vagina from where it passes down the urethra and into the bladder, showing the whole of the lower urinary tract. This is a normal, continent bitch.

b. In this example, vagino-urethrography has been used to demonstrate an ectopic ureter which is opening into the urethra rather than the bladder.

c. In this example, vagino-urethrography demonstrates that the bladder is positioned too far back in a bitch with urethral sphincter mechanism incompetence (compare with Fig. 12a).

incontinence surgery may be performed (see later section on '**Acquired urethral sphincter mechanism incompetence**'). In female animals with severe urethral hypoplasia, bladder neck reconstruction may be beneficial; however, this is mainly a problem of cats, rather than dogs.

Bladder hypoplasia – treatment of this condition may require anticholinergic drugs which may help to relax the bladder and allow an increase in filling before the urge to urinate occurs.

Pervious urachus – treatment involves surgical removal of the urachus.

Intersexuality – treatment involves surgical removal of the abnormal internal genitalia within which the urine is accumulating.

Congenital neurological conditions – unfortunately, there is often little which can be done and euthanasia of the animal is usually required because of the puppy's poor quality of life and secondary problems developing because of the paralysis. Depending on the site and severity of the condition causing it, this paralysis may affect the whole hind end of the animal (preventing normal walking, urination and defecation) or may predominantly affect the lower urinary tract, rectum and tail. If the condition is not too severe, some dedicated owners try to manage these animals but this requires nursing care every day and few owners have the skills and time do this. Most of these attempts fail in the long term for the reasons mentioned already.

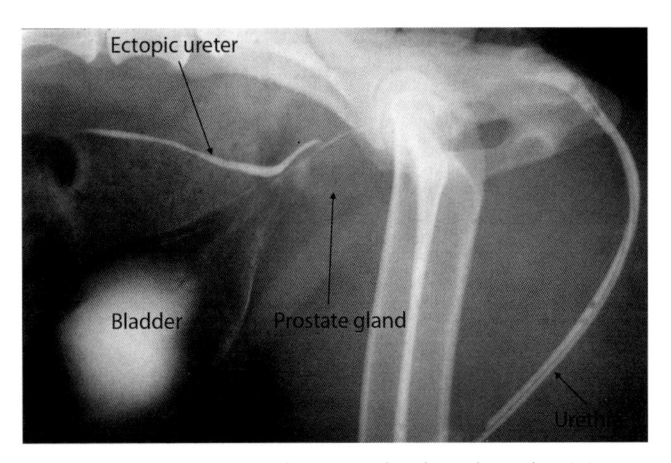

Fig. 13. In male dogs, contrast medium is introduced into the urethra via its opening on the tip of the penis. The contrast medium then passes up the long male urethra and into the bladder. The contrast medium in this dog is also passing into and demonstrating an ectopic ureter. The circular grey outline in the region where the ectopic ureter opens into the urethra is the prostate gland. This is often difficult to see, which is one of the reasons why veterinarians use ultrasonography as well as X-rays to visualise the prostate gland.

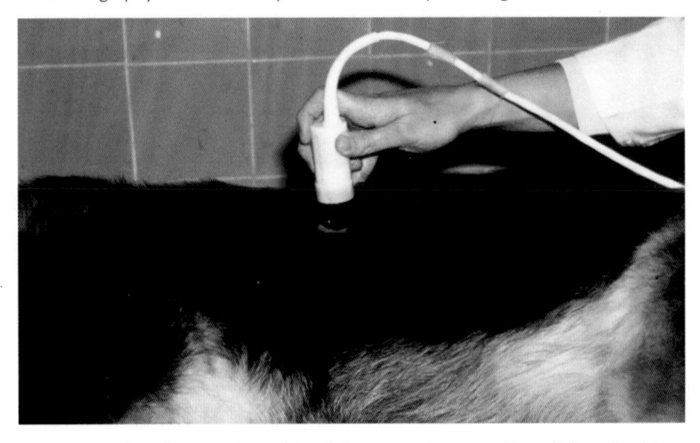

Fig. 14. Here the ultrasound machine is being used to examine a kidney in this German Shepherd dog.

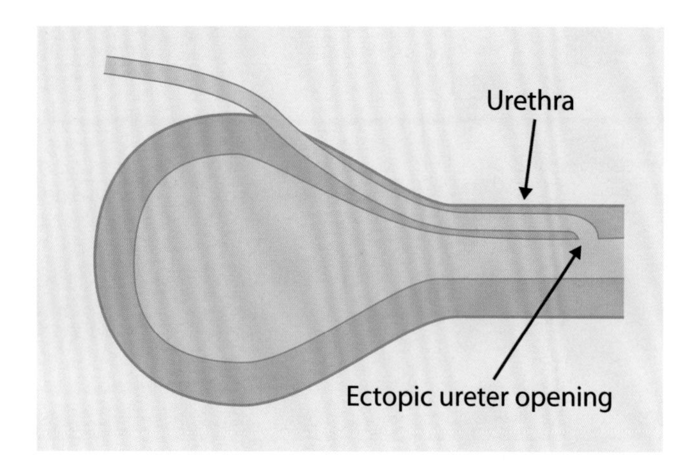

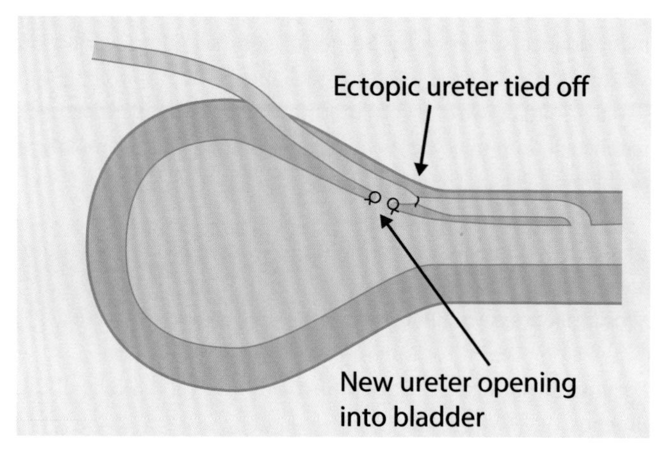

Fig. 15. Ectopic ureter transplantation. Note that the ectopic ureter usually enters the bladder wall normally but passes too far within the bladder and urethral walls to open ectopically, usually into the urethra, as shown in the left diagram. During the commonest surgical technique, a permanent opening is made between the ectopic ureter and the bladder and the ureter beyond this tied off (right diagram) or, sometimes, removed.

Adult incontinence

Acquired urethral sphincter mechanism incompetence – weight loss in an overweight dog is a simple thing which is worth trying. Acquired urethral sphincter mechanism incompetence can be treated medically or/and surgically. The three medical treatments currently licensed for the treatment of incontinent dogs are listed below. All of these drugs are aimed at increasing the tone of the smooth muscle in the urethral wall, thus tightening the sphincter:

- Alpha-adrenergic compounds such as phenylpropanolamine (Propalin, Vétoquinol; Urilin, Dechra Veterinary Products) and ephedrine (Enurace, Elanco Animal Health). Ephedrine may improve the bladder capacity through causing relaxation of the bladder muscles.
- The oestrogen estriol (Incurin, MSD Animal Health).

Affected spayed bitches may respond well to medical therapy but in some animals medication may become less effective over time. Some animals show no response to medication. Oestrogens sensitise the urethral smooth muscle to alpha-adrenergic stimulation and so a combination of oestrogen and alpha-adrenergic therapy may be useful and reduce the dose of each individual drug, lessening the chances of side effects (although none of the above drugs are licensed to be used in this combination).

The main options for surgical treatment are to attempt to:

- Increase urethral resistance – for example:
  - Peri-urethral surgical slings: this is a surgical technique where material is passed around the urethra to cause pressure on the urethra in an attempt to stop urine leakage.
  - Artificial sphincters: these are circular balloons which encircle the urethra and can be used to close it (when inflated). The balloon is emptied to allow urination. Artificial sphincters have not been used commonly in dogs
  - Intra-urethral injection of bulking agents: this involves injecting materials (usually collagen) into the wall of the urethra in an attempt to 'bulk' it up. The thicker urethral wall results in a narrower passage and thus reduces urine flow, hopefully resulting in a return of continence
- Increase urethral length, using bladder neck reconstruction techniques;
- Re-locate the bladder neck to an intra-abdominal position by means of either a colposuspension (a surgical technique whereby the vagina is stretched forward and attached to ligaments in front of the pelvis) or urethropexy (a surgical technique whereby the urethra is stitched to ligaments or the abdominal wall in front of the pelvis)

All of these techniques have been tried in dogs but by far the most popular techniques are colposuspension and intra-urethral injection of bulking agents since these have the same success rates as other methods but appear to have fewer complications.

The problem with techniques intended to increase urethral resistance is that they may make things worse by making an incontinent animal unable to urinate. Similarly, increasing urethral length carries potentially serious surgical risks and, in the author's view, should be reserved for animals with severe congenital urethral hypoplasia.

Colposuspension is intended to move the caudally positioned bladder neck of bitches with urethral sphincter mechanism incompetence to an intra-abdominal position so that increases in intra-abdominal pressure can act simultaneously on the bladder and urethra (*Fig.16*, page 26). Thus, any increase in intravesical pressure is counteracted by an increase in urethral resistance: a bit like squeezing a balloon (the bladder) and the neck of the balloon (the urethra) at the same time.

In comparison with the bitch, the condition in male dogs is less likely to respond to medical therapy. The pathophysiology of male urethral sphincter mechanism incompetence is poorly understood, making rational treatment difficult. Drugs used in its management include androgens, oestrogens and alpha-adrenergics. Of these, alpha-adrenergics (either alone or in combination with oestrogen) give the best results but, even then, more than half of treated dogs fail to respond to therapy. Androgens are, in the author's experience, ineffective. Attempts have been made surgically to relocate the intrapelvic bladder neck to an intra-abdominal position and intra-urethral injection of bulking agents have also been used. As with medical treatment, the impression in a limited number of cases is that surgical treatment alone of urethral sphincter mechanism incompetence is less successful in males than in bitches.

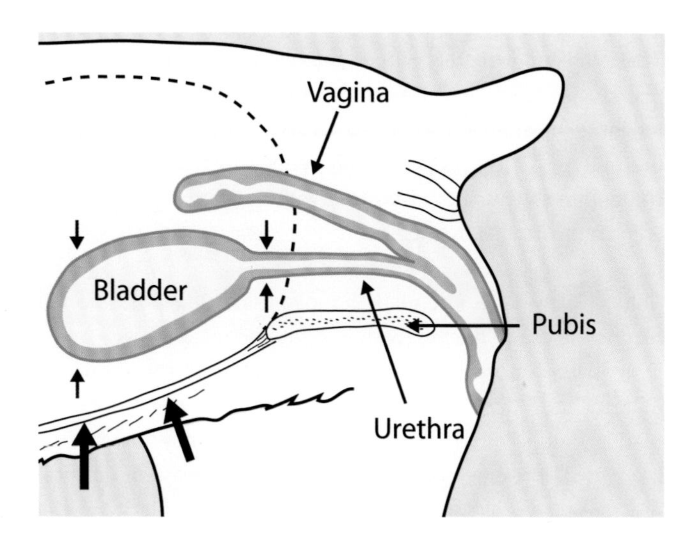

Prostatic disease – most prostatic diseases are benign and can be treated. By far the commonest condition is benign prostatic hyperplasia (the prostate becomes enlarged because of a hormone imbalance, usually in the oversexed young male dog!) and this responds to medical treatments aimed at counteracting the excessive (usually male) hormones or castration. Prostate cancer is not usually treatable and is a painful, progressive condition. In such cases, treatment is aimed at alleviating the discomfort and the urinary signs to improve the quality of life for the animal until the time when such quality is reduced to the level that euthanasia is the kindest thing to do.

Bladder neoplasia – if incontinence is associated with bladder cancer, the outlook is poor. By the time the animal exhibits signs which can be detected by the owner, the tumour is too far

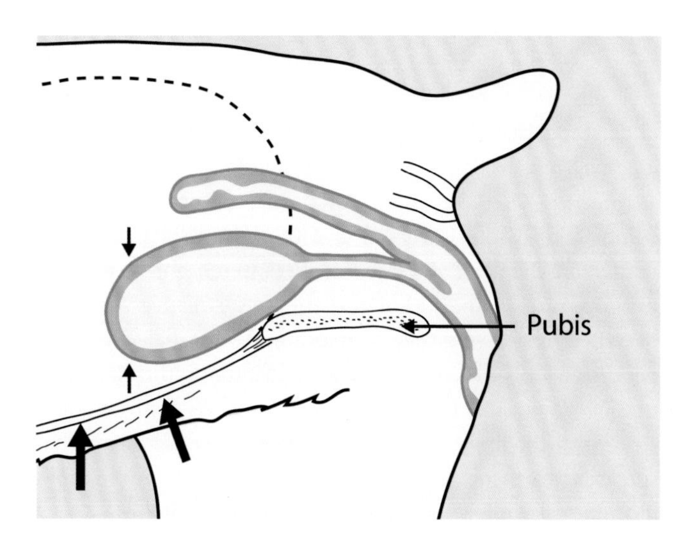

Fig. 16. The principle behind colposuspension. The bitch in the upper diagram has her bladder in a normal position, in front of the pelvis (the pubis is the floor of the pelvis). Thus both the bladder and the section of urethra adjacent to it are within the abdominal cavity. This means that when pressure is put on the abdomen (e.g. when the bitch lies down), represented by the large arrows, the resulting rise in pressure within the abdomen (small arrows) acts on both the bladder and the urethra. Thus any tendency for the increased pressure on the bladder to cause leakage is counteracted by the same pressure acting at the same time in the urethra, causing closure. Incontinence is therefore less likely to occur, if the urethral sphincter mechanism is incompetent.

Unfortunately for them, most bitches with urethral sphincter mechanism incompetence not only have an incompetent urethra but their bladders are also too far back, as shown on the lower diagram. This means that any increases in pressure within the abdomen are transmitted predominantly to the bladder only, making urine leakage more likely. Colposuspension is aimed at correcting this by moving the bladder forward into the abdomen so that pressures can act on both the bladder and urethra, hopefully cancelling each other out.

Compare these diagrams with Figs 12a and 12c on page 22.

advanced and/or in such a location that any surgery is too hazardous to other lower urinary tract organs or function and is rarely worthwhile. As with prostate cancer, treatment is aimed at alleviating the discomfort and the urinary signs to improve the quality of life for the animal until the time when such quality is reduced to the level that euthanasia is the kindest thing to do.

Ureterovaginal fistula – treatment is identical to that for congenital ectopic ureters although, sometimes, the adhesed ureter/vagina granuloma can be excised and the ureter ends re-joined.

Acquired neurological conditions – treatment is conservative (usually strict rest and anti-inflammatory/painkilling drugs) or surgical (spinal or neurological) depending on the cause, severity and duration of signs. In the case of tumours, little can usually be done and euthanasia may be required.

Overflow incontinence with chronic retention – treatment is aimed at removal of the obstruction. This is usually possible if the urethra is obstructed by a calculus (stone). In most cases, a calculus in the urethra is accompanied by more in the bladder and so attempts are usually made to return the urethral calculus to the bladder and then remove all calculi by one operation (a cystotomy). If the calculus is well and truly lodged in the urethra, it may have to be removed via a urethrotomy and the bladder stones removed separately, later. The calculi are then sent for analysis so that prophylactic measures can be instituted to prevent recurrence (these usually involve dietary changes and, sometimes, drugs). If the blockage cannot be removed (e.g. urethral cancer) then treatment is not possible. Some animals may have an improved quality of life by provision of urinary by-pass (usually a tube leading from the bladder out through the skin of the abdomen to drain urine from the bladder) along with drugs aimed at reducing the urgency and frequency associated with the tumour but these measures are not successful in all cases and, even if they are, this is merely short-term palliation and euthanasia will be required when the condition worsens to the extent that the dog has a poor quality of life.

Detrusor overactivity/instability – in cases secondary to other disorders, such as cystitis, treatment of the primary condition alone usually results in a return to continence. Animals with bladder hypoplasia and primary detrusor overactivity are much more difficult to treat but anticholinergic or smooth muscle anti-spasmodic drugs may be beneficial.

What outcomes can be expected for individual treatment methods?

Ectopic ureters – irrespective of the method of treatment, in the author's hands approximately 50% of animals are completely cured although in most of the remainder, the incontinence is markedly reduced. The response rate is not affected by the type of surgery performed and there is considerable discussion about why not all animals respond to surgery. Some possible reasons for no improvement after surgery are undiagnosed bilateral ectopic ureters, the presence of another cause of incontinence such as congenital urethral sphincter mechanism incompetence and/or bladder hypoplasia. In some instances, the reason for failure of response cannot be determined.

Congenital urethral sphincter mechanism incompetence -approximately half of affected bitches become continent following their first or second season (oestrus) and should thus **not** be spayed earlier! The prognosis in affected male dogs is guarded to poor, depending on the severity of the anatomical abnormalities. The author's impression is that urethral sphincter mechanism (congenital or acquired) in male dogs is more difficult to manage than in bitches.

Bladder hypoplasia – In most animals, following treatment of the main cause of incontinence (e.g. ectopic ureter), the bladder will develop to a normal size.

Pervious urachus –the outlook after surgery for this condition is excellent; surgery is usually curative unless another cause of incontinence is also present.

Intersexuality – most animals respond well to removal of the abnormal urine reservoir but in some there may also be congenital urethral sphincter mechanism incompetence present which may lead to a continuation of the incontinence.

Congenital neurological conditions – unfortunately, the outlook in these cases is usually poor.

Adult incontinence

Acquired urethral sphincter mechanism incompetence – the treatment of cases of urethral sphincter mechanism incompetence may be difficult and most therapies correct only one of the factors mentioned previously. It is unlikely, therefore, that any single method of treatment alone will cure 100% of animals treated. With any single method of treatment, 50% of the bitches treated will be cured in the long term, although most of the remainder are much less incontinent and may then respond to additional treatments using other therapies (e.g. a dog which fails to respond to surgery alone may then respond to medical therapy which it did not respond to before surgery). The response to medical or surgical management is not as good in male dogs. In both sexes, the condition may worsen as the animal gets older and incontinence can occasionally recur in later life in an animal which previously responded to treatment.

Prostate disease – the prognosis associated with most prostate conditions apart from cancer is good and the commonest condition, benign prostatic hyperplasia, is easily treatable, either with drugs or in the long term, if it keeps recurring, castration.

Bladder neoplasia – bladder cancers which are associated with incontinence as a sign are rarely treatable for the reasons given previously.

Ureterovaginal fistula – the outlook in these cases is good and a return to continence can be expected after successful surgery.

Acquired neurological conditions – the outlook in these cases depends on many factors and is often difficult to predict in the individual dog. Such factors as the cause of the paralysis, the duration and severity of the signs and the rate of progression of the signs are used to influence the veterinarian in giving a prognosis to the owner for his/her dog and the pros and cons of surgical versus non-surgical treatment.

Overflow incontinence with chronic retention – if the cause of the obstruction can be successfully removed before the bladder loses function, the prognosis in these cases is usually good. It is poorer if tumours are present or if the duration of the urinary retention means that permanent bladder damage has occurred secondary to the bladder distension. This is one of the reasons why animals that cannot urinate should be treated as emergencies.

Detrusor overactivity/instability – if a treatable cause can be detected, the outlook is usually good but it is poorer if a cause cannot be found and treatment can only be symptomatic.

What long-term care might be needed for a dog with incontinence?

Obviously, the aim is to determine the cause of the incontinence and treat it successfully. This is possible in the majority of incontinent dogs but what care may be required in those dogs that do not respond or are on long-term medical therapy?

Many owners manage their incontinent dogs very well with medications. For example, the bitch or male dog with urethral sphincter mechanism incompetence which responds well to medical management. These dogs are usually being treated with either alpha-adrenergic drugs such as phenylpropanolamine (Propalin, Vétoquinol; Urilin, Dechra Veterinary Products) or ephedrine (Enurace, Elanco Animal Health) or oestrogens such as estriol (Incurin, MSD Animal Health). Occasionally, alpha-adrenergics and oestrogens are used in combination, although they are not licensed for such combined use. There are potential side effects with these drugs although these appear to be extremely

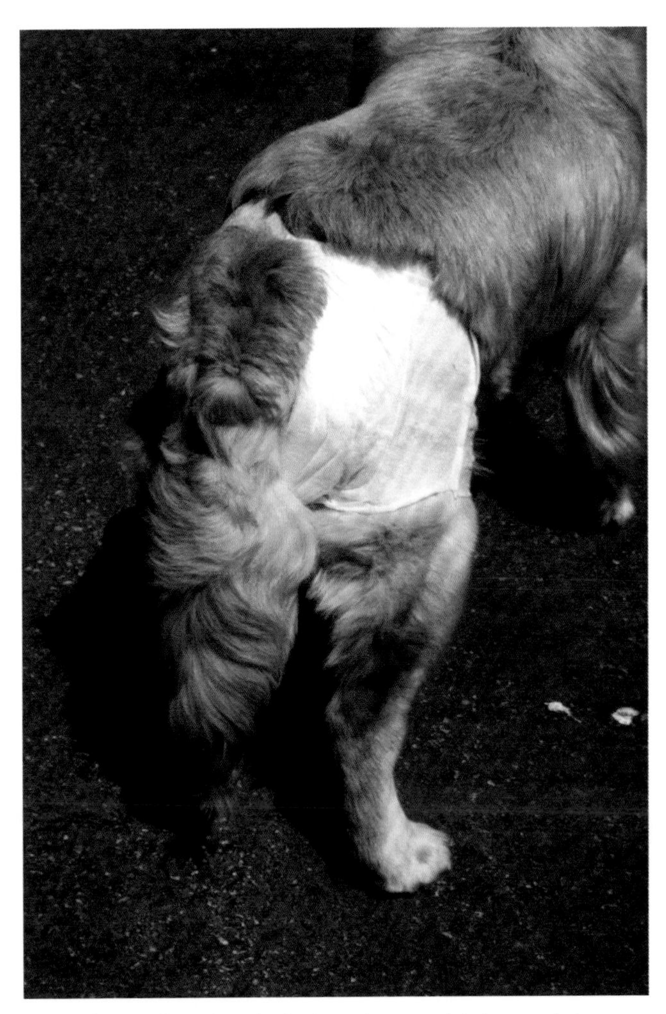

Fig. 17. The use of nappies and other incontinence pad devices may help to prevent contamination of the environment with urine but these require careful management to ensure the bitch's comfort and well-being.

rare. To make sure side effects are not developing, most veterinarians like to check animals being treated on a regular basis rather than merely handing out tablets without looking at the dog. Such checks need not be frequent but are a good idea to ensure that the dog is still responding as it should and no problems are developing. It is also an opportunity for the veterinarian to re-evaluate the treatments to see if any changes in drugs and/or dosages are required.

The long-term care of a dog with persistent incontinence is more of a problem. The aim of management in such cases is to minimise the effects of the incontinence on the dog's health (these effects vary from urine scalding of skin and secondary infections to the less common possibility of secondary kidney disease). Many owners manage the effects of the incontinence well by using barrier creams on the skin around the vulva or prepuce. Your veterinarian will be able to advise you on suitable creams to use although simple Vaseline is a good start. In dogs which may be at risk of secondary kidney problems or urinary tract infections, regular veterinary checks of the dog and also urine and, sometimes, blood laboratory work are required to spot problems which develop at an early stage and treat them accordingly. The other management problem is reducing the effects of the incontinence on the animal's home and other members of the household, human and animal. Apart from the effects of the urine in damaging carpets, bedding etc., there are potential health issues for the other inhabitants of the house. The urine contamination of the environment can be reduced by 'catching' the leaking urine. Thus many dogs are fitted with nappies, either human nappies adapted for the size, shape and sex of the dog or, in bitches, the strap-on 'pants' intended for bitches in season with a human incontinence pad inserted inside (*Fig. 17,* page 29). Whilst these methods can work, they require a lot of owner dedication. The nappy has to be removed when the dog is walked to allow it to urinate normally. Frequent nappy changes are required. At each change the area of the dog where urine has been leaking has to be washed and barrier cream applied. This is not easy and some owners find they cannot cope with this management in the long term. That and their feeling that the dog has a poor quality of life sometimes results in them requesting euthanasia of the animal. Other owners are able to devote this major time commitment to their dog and, if the dog is accepting of the changes required (nappies, washing, confinement in one part of the house etc.) and has a good quality of life, continue to manage their dogs this way. The wearing of nappies may make the dog more susceptible to skin and urinary tract infections (hence the need for cleanliness when using these) and it is prudent to allow your veterinarian to re-examine your dog from time to time (and helpful if you take a fresh urine sample in with you when you do) to ensure this is not happening.

Interestingly, in multi-dog households, the other dogs may assist in the management! They are sometimes prepared to lick and clean the affected dog and some incontinent dogs learn to 'request' this service from them. The dogs doing the cleaning appear to suffer no ill effects as a result of providing this assistance.

Most of the veterinary checks mentioned above probably only need performing about every three months but obviously these should be sooner if the owner thinks a problem might be developing.

Fliss: an incontinent Golden Retriever puppy and her treatment for ectopic ureter

Fliss was a Golden Retriever puppy bred by her owner Jill. Jill had bred several litters of Golden Retrievers previously with no problems in any of the puppies. Fliss was the runt of the litter and had a curious, slightly hoarse bark. More importantly, she was incontinent, leaking urine continuously. Apart from Fliss' littermates, Jill had four other adult Goldies in her house and all dogs had 'full access' to all the furniture. The dogs would usually sleep together in various combinations. This meant that, before long, not only did Fliss stink of urine but so did her littermates and her adult canine housemates, as well as the furniture. Jill managed this by frequent bathing of Fliss and all the other dogs in the house and by the use of a pair of strap-on pants and incontinence pads on Fliss. By twelve weeks of age, all Fliss' littermates had gone to good homes but Jill, quite rightly, would not pass the problem of an incontinent dog on to a new owner. When Fliss was four months old, Jill therefore had her incontinence investigated and this showed that Fliss had an ectopic ureter. Although she was aware that surgery for this condition is not always successful, Jill opted to have Fliss treated. Fliss' ectopic ureter was transplanted into her bladder using the technique described previously. Fortunately, she responded well to surgery and the incontinence resolved, allowing her to go to a good home without wearing the pants! Seven years later, she is still living with the same loving family and remains 'bone dry'.

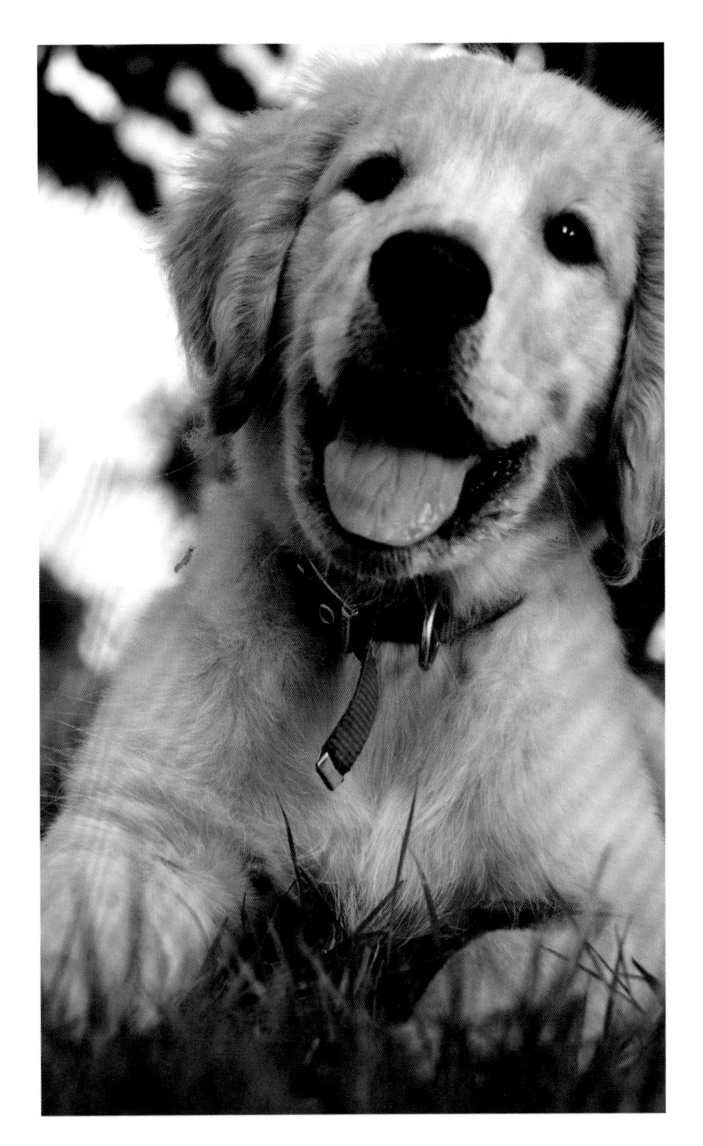

Tara: an incontinent adult Doberman pinscher and her treatment for urethral sphincter mechanism incompetence

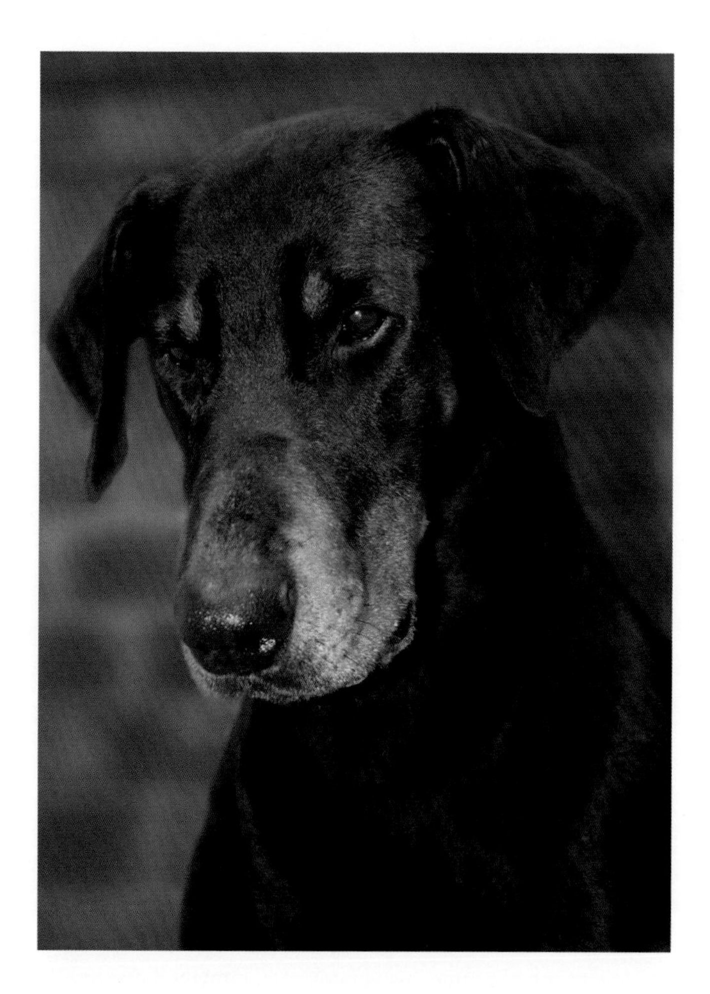

Tara was a seven year old spayed Doberman pinscher bitch. She had developed urinary incontinence two years previously. Urine leakage only occurred when she was lying down and relaxed and, initially, was only slight. She would leak only drops of urine once or twice monthly. At that stage, she was not treated because her owners felt they could tolerate this degree of leakage. However, over the next twelve months, the incontinence gradually worsened to the extent that Tara was leaking pools of urine every day. Medical treatments tried were phenylpropanolamine (an alpha-adrenergic), estriol (an oestrogen) and the combination of phenylpropanolamine and estriol but there was no response to any of these. Investigation of her incontinence confirmed that it was due to urethral sphincter mechanism incompetence and in view of the lack of response to medical therapy, the owners opted for surgical treatment. A colposuspension was performed. The owners reported that she was 90% better – i.e. she was dry most of the time but did still exhibit occasional incontinence. It was suggested that, despite the previous poor response, they should try medical treatment again. Tara was therefore put back onto phenylpropanolamine therapy and on this occasion she responded and became continent. This case is an illustration that one form of treatment (medical or surgical) may not be sufficient alone to resolve the incontinence. In Tara's case, a combination of surgical and medical treatment resolved the problem. This case also demonstrates that animals that do not respond to medical treatment before surgery may do so afterwards if a degree of incontinence persists. So the fact that an incontinent bitch does not respond to medical treatment before surgery should not prevent such treatment being tried again if surgery fails to resolve the incontinence.

SECTION 4 | discussing your dog's health with your veterinarian

As mentioned previously, a good history is very useful in incontinence cases. It is very helpful, therefore, if when you consult your veterinarian about your dog's incontinence, you have the relevant information to hand. So, be prepared to answer the following questions (let's assume your veterinarian hasn't seen your dog previously); some of these questions may be self-evident:

- What is your dog's name?
- How old is he/she?
- What sex is he/she?
- When did you first notice the incontinence?
- Has the incontinence got worse over time (increased volumes of urine leakage and/or increased frequency of bouts of incontinence)?
- As well as leaking urine, does your dog also pass urine normally when taken for walks, allowed in the garden etc.?
- Does urine leakage occur every day or do you have 'wet' and 'dry' days?
- When does urine leakage occur? Is it worse when your dog is lying down and relaxed or is the urine leakage the same all the time?
- How extensive is the leakage of urine? Does your dog leave puddles of urine where it has been lying? Is the hair around your dog's vulva or prepuce always wet with urine?
- Does your dog appear to be aware of the urine leakage?
- Does incontinence only occur when your dog gets excited – e.g. urinates when he/she first greets you?
- Is your dog neutered? If so, when was he/she neutered? Was this before or after the first season? Did the incontinence begin after your dog was neutered or was it present prior to that?
- Do you notice any other urinary signs, for example urinary urgency, increased frequency, difficulty in passing urine or passing blood in the urine?
- Is your dog otherwise well or is he/she off colour and not eating as well as you would expect?
- Does your dog drink excessively? It may be helpful to measure how much water your dog is drinking over a 24 hour period and take this information to your veterinarian. For example, a measured amount of water (A) is placed in the bowl. 24 hours later, the amount of water remaining is measured (B) and the total consumed calculated (A-B). In households where there are multiple animals, it can be difficult to

measure water consumption for one dog but a total household water consumption may still be helpful and offers something that can be monitored over time – this is especially relevant in cases where there is an abnormal thirst for example due to an illness such as diabetes mellitus ('sugar diabetes').

- Is your dog losing weight?

- Have you noticed any deterioration in your dog's ability to walk normally, especially related to the back legs?

- Does your dog pass faeces normally (i.e. without straining and/or the presence of blood)?

The information in this section is mainly relevant to owners of dogs in the extremely rare situation where the incontinence is associated with cancer and where decisions may have to be made regarding euthanasia.

Knowing when to say goodbye

How long has my dog got before euthanasia is required and how will I know when it is time?

This is difficult and varies enormously from animal to animal. It is rare, in our pets, for the cancer to actually kill the dog and, if we wait for it to do so, the animal's quality of life by then will be awful. In some dogs with cancer, the condition can be managed and the animal's quality of life maintained for quite some time until it deteriorates to a point where euthanasia is the only option. In other dogs this period is sadly very short. One of the problems is that, living with your pet, it is often difficult to judge deterioration. Apart from your emotional involvement with your dog, deterioration can be quite subtle and difficult to discern on a day-to-day basis. A useful thing to do is to allow your veterinarian to examine your dog regularly. Since he/she will not be seeing your pet as often as you do, he/she may pick up on a deterioration which you might have missed. Most sensible owners are more concerned about 'leaving things too long'. That is, much as they love their dog and will miss it terribly, they don't want to prolong life to the extent that the animal's quality of life was really poor towards the end and, with the benefit of hindsight, they wish they had made the decision for euthanasia sooner. Please let your veterinarian help you with this decision and guide you as to when the time is right to allow your pet to die peacefully.

What does euthanasia involve?

Euthanasia usually involves your veterinarian giving your dog an injection of a concentrated anaesthetic drug intravenously (directly into a vein). In effect, this is an anaesthetic overdose and rapidly results in your dog losing consciousness and then dying shortly afterwards. The only pain involved is that of the injection, which is usually minimal. In some dogs, immediately after death, there appear to be one or two breathing movements. This is a reflex action and does not mean that the dog is still alive or distressed. Most dogs are euthanased at the veterinary hospital, since expert nursing help is at hand to minimise handling stress during this procedure although most veterinarians are happy to come to the owners home to do this, if desired. Most veterinarians are also very happy for the owner to stay with their dog and, in many cases, give the dog a last cuddle while this is taking place. Although you will feel sad that you have had to have your dog euthanased, please try to remember that this is the last kind thing you can do for your pet.

What happens to my dog's body after it dies or is euthanased?

There are two main options:

- You could bury your dog's body at home.
- Your veterinarian can arrange for your dog's body to be cremated. In the case of an individual cremation, your dog's ashes can be returned to you for burial or scattering in their favourite place.

It is useful to discuss euthanasia of your dog and the options for dealing with the body with your veterinarian while your dog is still well. While this may seem a little macabre, you will be thinking more clearly and will be more able to make decisions than you will on the day when euthanasia is finally required.

How to cope with losing your dog

Is there support available to me in my grief?

Losing a treasured dog is like losing any other member of the family. There are various stages in the grieving process and you are likely to go through some, if not all, of these. They include denial, anger, guilt, depression and finally acceptance. Once your dog has been diagnosed with an incurable condition such as cancer, you may experience some of these feelings even while your pet is still alive.

The best support is obtained from family and friends, especially those who have owned pets and have been through a similar loss themselves. You are likely to have seen a lot of your veterinarian and the nurses at the veterinary practice and built up a strong rapport if not friendship with them and they should also be able to offer you support. They may also be able to direct you to local support groups. There is a UK helpline dedicated to pet bereavement counselling, the Pet Bereavement Support Service (PBSS). The contact telephone number is 0800 096 6606 and is manned from 8.30am to 8.30pm daily. All calls are free and confidential and the PBSS also offers an e-mail support service (**pbssmail@bluecross.org.uk**). More information can be found on-line at: **http://www.bluecross.org.uk/web/site/AboutUs/PetBereavement/ContactingPBSS.asp**

Are my other dog(s) likely to grieve?

Although grieving is a very human emotion, dogs can also show 'grief' at the loss of a canine companion. The response is variable. Some dogs appear unaffected by the loss and others may seem happier now that they are on their own. However, others may exhibit signs such as restlessness and sleeping less, not eating as much, appearing to search for their lost companion, barking more or appearing more miserable in general than usual. These signs usually settle down within six months but can last a year.

In many ways, you can support your remaining dog in the same way that you would support a human friend by:

- Keeping to the same routines in the home.
- Continue to give your dog the love and attention you always have, if anything even more so during this mourning period for you both.
- Encouraging your dog to eat and exercise as usual, including going on the same walks you always did when the other dog was alive.
- Some owners think replacing the dog that has died/been put to sleep may help the remaining dog to obtain a new lease of life and this is true in many cases. However, not all dogs respond in this way and it is prudent to wait for a few months before introducing a new dog. In the meantime, it may be helpful to 'dog-sit' a friend's dog in your house for a day or so to see how your remaining dog responds to new company

and to get an impression if introducing a new dog into the household might or might not be a good idea.

Further Reading

For those with a more scientific interest in this subject and who would like to explore it in more depth, here are some references you may wish to look at. Please read all of these critically, especially those relating to treatments of incontinence. Things to look out for are how many animals received the treatment and over how long a period after surgery or while on medication were the dogs followed up for – you as an owner need to know the effectiveness of treatment in a significant number of dogs over a period of years, rather than weeks or months!

AARON, A., EGGLETON, E., POWER, C. & HOLT, P.E. (1996) *Urethral sphincter mechanism incompetence in male dogs: a retrospective analysis of 54 cases. Veterinary Record 139, 542-546.*

ATALAN, G. HOLT, P.E. & BARR, F.J. (1998) *Ultrasonographic assessment of bladder neck mobility in continent bitches and bitches with urinary incontinence attributable to urethral sphincter mechanism incompetence. American Journal of Veterinary Research, 59, 673-679.*

BACON, N.J., ONI, O. & WHITE, R.A.S. (2002) *Treatment of urethral sphincter mechanism incompetence in 11 bitches with a sustained-release formulation of phenylpropanolamine hydrochloride. Veterinary Record 151, 373-376.*

BARTH, A., REICHLER, I.M., HUBLER, M., HASSIG, M. & ARNOLD, S. (2005) *Evaluation of long-term effects of endoscopic injection of collagen into the urethral submucosa for treatment of urethral sphincter mechanism incompetence in female dogs: 40 cases (1993-2000). Journal of the American Veterinary Medical Association 226, 73-76.*

DEAN, P.W., NOVOTNY, M.J. & O'BRIEN, D.P. (1989) *Prosthetic sphincter for urinary incontinence: results in three cases. Journal of the American Animal Hospital Association, 25, 447-454.*

HOLT, P.E. (1985) *Urinary incontinence in the bitch due to sphincter mechanism incompetence: prevalence in referred dogs and retrospective analysis of sixty cases. Journal of Small Animal Practice, 26, 181-190.*

HOLT, P.E. (1985) *Importance of urethral length, bladder neck position and vestibulovaginal stenosis in sphincter mechanism incompetence in the incontinent bitch. Research in Veterinary Science, 39, 364-372*

HOLT, P.E. (1990) *Urinary incontinence in dogs and cats. Veterinary Record 127, 347-350.*

HOLT, P.E. (1990) *Long-term evaluation of colposuspension in the treatment of urinary incontinence due to incompetence of the urethral sphincter mechanism in the bitch. Veterinary Record, 127, 537-542.*

HOLT, P.E. (1993) *Surgical management of congenital urethral sphincter mechanism incompetence in eight female cats and a bitch. Veterinary Surgery, 22, 98-104.*

HOLT, P.E. (2000) FECAVA LECTURE. *Investigation and therapy of incontinent animals. European Journal of Companion Animal Practice 10, 111-116.*

HOLT, P.E. & THRUSFIELD, M.V. (1993) *Association in bitches between breed, size, neutering and docking, and acquired urinary incontinence due to incompetence of the urethral sphincter mechanism. Veterinary Record, 133, 177-180.*

HOLT, P.E. & JONES, A. (2000) *In vitro study of the significance of bladder neck position in incontinent bitches. Veterinary Record 146,437-439.*

HOLT, P.E., COE, R.J. & HOTSTON MOORE, A. (2005) *Prostatopexy as a treatment for urethral sphincter mechanism incompetence in male dogs. Journal of Small Animal Practice 46, 567-570.*

MANDIGERS, P.J.J. & NELL, T. (2001) *Treatment of bitches with acquired urinary incontinence with oestriol. Veterinary Record 149, 764-767.*

MARCHEVSKY, A.M., EDWARDS, G.A., LAVELLE, R.B. & ROBERTSON, I.D. (1999) *Colposuspension in 60 bitches with incompetence of the urethral sphincter mechanism. Australian Veterinary Practititioner 29, 2.*

MASSAT, B.J., GREGORY, C.R., LING, G.V. CARDINET, G.H. & LEWIS, E.L. (1993) *Cystourethropexy to correct refractory urinary incontinence due to urethral sphincter mechanism incompetence. Preliminary results in ten bitches. Veterinary Surgery 22, 260-268.*

MUIR, P., GOLDSMID, S.E. & BELLENGER, C.R. (1994) *Management of urinary incontinence in five bitches with incompetence of the urethral sphincter mechanism by colposuspension and a modified sling urethroplasty. Veterinary Record 134, 38-41.*

NICKEL, R.F., WIEGAND, U. & VAN DEN BROM, W.E. (1998) *Evaluation of a transpelvic sling procedure with and without colposuspension for treatment of female dogs with refractory urethral sphincter mechanism incompetence. Veterinary Surgery 27, 94-104.*

POWER, S.C., EGGLETON, K.E., AARON, A,J., HOLT, P.E. & CRIPPS, P.J. (1998) *Urethral sphincter mechanism incompetence in the male dog: importance of bladder neck position, proximal urethral length and castration. Journal of Small Animal Practice 39, 69-72.*

RAWLINGS, C.A., BARSANTI, J.A., MAHAFFEY, M.B. & BEMENT, S. (2001) *Evaluation of colposuspension for treatment of incontinence in spayed female dogs. Journal of the American Veterinary Medical Association 219, 770-775.*

RICHTER, K.P. & LING, G.V. (1985) *Clinical response and urethral pressure profile changes after phenylpropanolamine in dogs with primary sphincter incompetence. Journal of the American Veterinary Medical Association 187, 605-611.*

SALOMON, J.F., COTARD, J.P. & VIGUIER, E. (2002) *Management of urethral sphincter mechanism incompetence in a male dog with laparoscopic-guided deferentopexy. Journal of Small Animal Practice 43, 501-505.*

SCOTT, L., LEDDY, M., BERNAY, F. & DAVOT, J.L. (2002) *Evaluation of phenylpropanolamine in the treatment of urethral sphincter mechanism incompetence in the bitch. Journal of Small Animal Practice 43, 493-496.*

THRUSFIELD, M.V., MUIRHEAD, R.H. & HOLT, P.E. (1998) *Acquired urinary incontinence in bitches: its incidence and relationship to neutering practices. Journal of Small Animal Practice 39, 559-566.*

WEBER, U. T., ARNOLD, S., HUBLER, M. & KUPPER, J.R. (1997) *Surgical treatment of male dogs with urinary incontinence due to urethral sphincter mechanism incompetence. Veterinary Surgery 26, 51-56.*

WHITE, R.A.S. & POMEROY, C.J. (1989) *Phenylpropanolamine: an a-adrenergic agent for the management of urinary incontinence in the bitch associated with urethral sphincter mechanism incompetence. Veterinary Record 125, 478-480.*

WHITE, R.N. (2001) *Urethropexy for the management of urethral sphincter mechanism incompetence in the bitch. Journal of Small Animal Practice 42, 481-486.*

Glossary of terms used by veterinarians

Term	Definition
Abdomen	The cavity behind the chest cavity of the dog and which contains the urinary tract, gastro-intestinal tract and other internal organs such as the liver.
Acquired urethral sphincter mechanism incompetence	Incompetence of the urethral sphincter mechanism which develops later in life in a dog which was previously continent.
Alpha-adrenergic	A drug which stimulates specific receptors (the alpha receptors) of the sympathetic nervous system.
Androgens	Male sex hormones (usually testosterone). Testosterone is produced naturally by the testes.
Anticholinergic	A drug which dampens down the activity of the parasympathetic system, used in the urinary tract to suppress unstable bladder contractions.
Artefacts	This is where misleading abnormalities appear to be present on a test or X-ray when in fact they are not real.
Artificial sphincters	These are circular balloons which encircle the urethra and can be used to close it (when inflated). To allow urination, the balloon is emptied. They have been used rarely in dogs.
Bilateral	This means that both sides are affected. For example in a dog with bilateral ectopic ureters, both the right and left ureter bypass the bladder to open lower down the urinary tract.
Biopsy	A small sample taken, and examined microscopically, to try to determine the nature of a mass or to look for abnormalities.
Bulking agents	These are materials (usually collagen) which are injected into the wall of the urethra in an attempt to 'bulk' it up. The thicker urethral wall results in a narrower passage and thus reduces urine flow, hopefully to a level resulting in a return to continence.
Calculi	Stones, usually found in the urinary tract. The single term is 'calculus'.
Cancer	Malignant tumour which not only grows where it originally started, but can also invade adjacent tissues and spread (metastasise) to other parts of the body. Common sites for metastasis include the lungs and liver. Left untreated, most cancers will ultimately cause the death of the dog.
Caudally	Towards the rear (tail) end of the animal.

Term	Definition
Colposuspension	A technique where the vagina is stretched forward and attached to ligaments in front of the pelvis. Since the urethra is attached to the vagina, it is also moved forward and this operation is used to move a bladder neck which is too far back, forward into the abdomen.
Congenital	A problem that the animal is born with, usually due to a problem of normal development of the foetus in the womb.
Contrast radiography	An X-ray examination where a liquid which shows up on X-ray films is used to outline organs which would be difficult to see otherwise.
CT	Computerised Tomography – a scanning technique where multiple X-ray images are taken to build up a picture of internal organs.
Cystitis	Inflammation of the bladder, usually associated with bacterial urinary tract infections in dogs.
Cystometric	Urodynamic measurements within the urinary bladder.
Cystotomy	An operation where the bladder is opened up (e.g. to remove calculi).
Detrusor	Relating to the urinary bladder.
Detrusor overactivity/ instability	Uncontrolled bladder contractions where the cause is unclear (overactivity) or due to causes other than neurological problems (instability).
Detrusor reflex	The emptying of the bladder which occurs when it is full. After bladder training, dogs are usually able to exert control over this reflex.
Dilated/dilatation	Dilated means a hollow organ is enlarged because it contains too much fluid or gas. For example 'dilated ureter' means the ureter is enlarged because too much urine is accumulating in it. A dilatation is a dilated portion of a hollow organ.
Diverticula	The plural of diverticulum which means an out-pouching from a hollow organ.
Dysuria	Usually taken to mean difficulty in passing urine.
Ectopic ureter/s	This is where the ureter fails to open normally into the bladder but bypasses it and opens lower down the urinary tract, leading to incontinence. Also referred to as ureteral ectopia.

Term	Definition
Endoscope	An instrument used for looking inside the animal, usually a flexible, fibre-optic device or video-endoscope.
Euthanasia	The humane termination of an animals life. Also referred to as 'putting to sleep'.
Excised	Cut out.
Fistula	An abnormal communication between two hollow organs.
Genitalia	Genital or sex organs.
Granuloma	A mass of chronically inflamed tissue. Chronic means present for a long time (usually one month or longer).
Haematuria	The presence of blood in the urine.
Histopathological	Examination of tissues under a microscope.
Hydronephrosis	Abnormal dilation of the collecting area in the kidney (the renal pelvis) with urine.
Hypoplasia	Hypoplasia of an organ is where the organ has failed to develop to its normal size.
Hydro-ureter	Abnormal dilation of the ureter with urine.
Intersexuality	Where both male and female sex organs are present in the same animal.
Intervertebral disc prolapse	This is where the padding material (the disc) between the bones of the spine (the vertebrae) moves and may impinge on the nerves within the spine.
Intra-abdominal	Within the abdomen.
Intramural	Literally, within the wall.
Intrapelvic	Within the canal of the pelvis.
Intravesical	Within the bladder.
Intravesical stomatisation	A technique used to treat ectopic ureter where a new opening is made from the ureter into the bladder.

Term	Definition
Intravenous urography	A technique where a liquid which shows up on X-rays is injected into a vein, passes round the circulation and is excreted by the kidneys. This is useful for outlining the kidneys and ureters.
Kidney	This is a bean-shaped organ found in the front part of the abdomen. There are two kidneys, a left and a right.
Ligation	This means tying off – e.g. when a blood vessel has suture material passed around it and is tied to stop it bleeding.
Lower urinary tract	The ureters, bladder and urethra
Mammary	Relating to the breasts.
MRI	Magnetic Resonance Imaging – a method of scanning the body to look for abnormalities in internal organs and bones.
Neoplasia	Another word for tumours/abnormal growths. See entry for cancer.
Neurological	Relating to the nervous system.
Neuromuscular	Relating to the function of muscles and their nerve supply.
Nocturia	Urinating overnight (usually in the house).
Oestrogen/s	Female sex hormones produced naturally by the ovaries. High levels of oestrogens are present when a bitch is in season.
Oestrus	The term used when a bitch is in season.
Palliation	The use of methods to improve health and quality of life in animals with untreatable conditions.
Paraplegia	Paralysis of the back legs.
Pathophysiology	The abnormalities which might lead to or predispose to a particular condition.
Perineum	The small area of skin between the anus and the vulva in the female or between the anus and the scrotum in the male dog

Term	Definition
Peri-urethral surgical sling	A technique where material is passed around the urethra, usually to cause pressure on the urethra in an attempt to eliminate urine leakage. The use of slings without tension (as used in incontinent women) is just being introduced into veterinary surgery and we must await the results obtained with these.
Pervious urachus	Pervious urachus is where a communication (the urachus), which is present in the foetus, between the bladder and the umbilicus (navel) fails to close before birth.
Pituitary gland	A gland on the floor of the brain which produces hormones which control the secretion of hormones from other glands in the body.
Prepuce	The sheath around the male dog's penis.
Prognosis	The outlook associated with treating a condition. For example, a good prognosis means the animal is likely to do well.
Prophylactic	Preventative.
Prostatic disease/s	Disease/s of the prostate gland which encircles the urethra near where it joins the bladder of male dogs.
Pyelonephritis	Infection of the kidney affecting the collecting area (renal pelvis) as well as the kidney itself.
Pyometra	A severe infection of the womb in dogs.
Scalding/scalded	Also known as 'urine burn', inflammation of the perineum, and sometimes the hindlegs, by urine. Urine scalding can occur as a consequence of urinary incontinence or if a dog is unable to assume normal posture when urinating (for example if paralysed). Prolonged contact between urine and skin can result in severe inflammation. Secondary infection of the dermatitis may also occur.
Smooth muscle	Muscle over which the animal has no voluntary control.
Sphincter	This is a (usually) circular muscle which is used to regulate flow from one organ into another or to the outside. Although in the past people talked about a 'bladder sphincter' which controls urine outflow from the bladder, we now know it is not quite as simple as that (see Section 2)!
Stoma	A permanent opening made between two hollow organs or a hollow organ and the outside of the body.

Term	Definition
Striated muscle	Muscle over which the animal has voluntary control (so called because stripes are visible in this muscle under a microscope).
Ultrasonography	A technique using ultrasonic sound waves to obtain a picture of internal organs.
Umbilicus	The navel or belly button.
Ureter/s	This is the fine tube that transports urine from the kidney to the bladder. There are two ureters – one from each kidney to the bladder.
Ureteral ectopia	This means the same as 'ectopic ureter'.
Ureterovaginal fistula	An abnormal communication (a fistula) between a ureter and the vagina.
Urethra	The tube which transports urine from the bladder to the outside.
Urethral hypoplasia	Where the animal is born with a urethra which is too short.
Urethral pressure profilometry	A urodynamic test intended to measure the tone in the urethral wall.
Urethral sphincter mechanism	The term used to summarise the forces acting in the urethra to keep the urethra closed and maintain continence.
Urethral sphincter mechanism incompetence	Used to describe the situation where the urethral tone is poor, allowing urine to leak out and thus leading to incontinence.
Urethrocystography	A technique where a liquid which shows up white on X-rays is used to outline the urethra and bladder. Usually used in male dogs.
Urethropexy	A technique where the urethra is sutured to ligaments or the abdominal wall in front of the pelvis. This is used to move a bladder neck which is too far back, forward into the abdomen.
Urethrotomy	An operation where the urethra is opened up (usually to remove stones).
Urinary bladder	This is the muscular sac within which urine is stored before being expelled when the dog urinates.
Urinary incontinence	Passive leakage of urine between normal urinations.

Term	Definition
Urodynamic investigations	Investigations which involve measuring the pressures in the urinary tract organs.
Vagina	The tube leading from the uterus to the outside in female animals.
Vagino-urethrography	A technique where a liquid which shows up on X-rays is introduced into the vagina of bitches to outline the vagina, urethra and bladder.
Vascular	Relating to the blood vessels.
Vesicovaginal fistulation	An abnormal communication (a fistula) between the bladder and vagina.
Vulva	The opening of the vagina.